EVIDENCE-BASED
MEDICINE

How to Practice and Teach EBM

Dedications

This book is dedicated to Kilgore Trout, the right stuff, crossroads, Bubbles & Squeak, and all the chips.

For Churchill Livingstone:

Commissioning Editor: Michael Parkinson
Project Development Manager: Janice Urquhart
Project Manager: Nancy Arnott
Design direction: Judith Wright
Page makeup: Kate Walshaw
Illustrated by: Robert Britton

EVIDENCE-BASED MEDICINE

How to Practice and Teach EBM

David L. Sackett
Director, Trout Research and Conference Centre, Irish Lake, Ontario, Canada

Sharon E. Straus
Consultant General Physician, University Health Network,
Mount Sinai Hospital, University of Toronto, Toronto, Ontario, Canada

W. Scott Richardson
Director, Three Owl Learning Institute and Associate Professor of Medicine,
Wright State University School of Medicine, Dayton, Ohio, USA

William Rosenberg
Senior Lecturer in Medicine and Honorary Consultant Physician,
University of Southampton, Southampton General Hospital,
Southampton, UK

R. Brian Haynes
Professor of Clinical Epidemiology and Medicine, McMaster University,
Hamilton, Ontario, Canada

SECOND EDITION

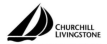
CHURCHILL
LIVINGSTONE

EDINBURGH LONDON NEW YORK PHILADELPHIA ST LOUIS SYDNEY TORONTO 2000

CHURCHILL LIVINGSTONE
An imprint of Harcourt Publishers Limited

© David L. Sackett, Sharon E. Straus, W. Scott Richardson,
William Rosenberg and R. Brian Haynes 2000

 is a registered trade mark of Harcourt Publishers Limited

The right of David L. Sackett, Sharon E. Straus, W. Scott Richardson,
William Rosenberg and R. Brian Haynes to be identified as authors
of this work has been asserted by them in accordance with the
Copyright, Designs and Patents Act 1988.

First published 1997
This edition 2000
Reprinted 2000 (three times)
Reprinted 2001

ISBN 0 443 06240 4

British Library Cataloguing in Publication Data
A catalogue record for this book is available from the British Library.

Library of Congress Cataloging in Publication Data
A catalog record for this book is available from the Library of Congress.

Medical knowledge is constantly changing. As new information becomes
available, changes in treatment, procedures, equipment and the use of
drugs become necessary. The authors and the publishers have, as far as
it is possible, taken care to ensure that the information given in this text is
accurate and up to date. However, readers are strongly advised to confirm
that the information, especially with regard to drug usage, complies with
current legislation and standards of practice.

The
publisher's
policy is to use
**paper manufactured
from sustainable forests**

Printed in China

Resources that accompany this text

The chapters and appendices that comprise this book constitute a traditional way of presenting our ideas about EBM. Although it may suffice for some of you, we think our book suffers from three major short-comings: First, its clinical examples are constricted by the narrow clinical perspective of the general physicians who wrote it; readers from other branches of medicine, and especially from other health professions, face the frustrating (but hopefully fulfilling) task of transposing the lessons to their own patients and settings. Second, the descriptions of evidence-sources are restricted by the limits of print space (and the size of your pockets!). Finally, this book is stuck in amber, and parts of it (written in early 1999) will be out-of-date by the time it appears in print (in late 1999).

We've decided to try to overcome these deficiencies by employing some of the same innovations in information packaging (the accompanying CD) and communication (the book's website) that have made the modern practice of EBM possible.

The accompanying compact disk

The CD tucked inside the cover of this book attacks the first and second of its shortcomings. First, it contains *clinical examples, critical appraisals, and background papers from 14 other health disciplines*. As a result, health professionals from these other disciplines can substitute them for the examples and appraisals in this book and much more easily integrate its message into their own clinical practice. Second, it contains *extended descriptions (including sample web pages) of several current evidence sources* regularly consulted by the authors of this book.

To install from Windows

1. Insert the EBM CD-ROM in your computer's CD-ROM drive
2. Choose Run from Start menu (File menu for Windows 3.1)
3. Type d:\setup.exe (if your CD is assigned to a letter other than D, use the correct letter in the command line)
4. Follow the on screen instructions.

To install from Macintosh

1. Insert the EBM CD-ROM in your computer's CD-ROM drive
2. Double-click the 'Install EBM' icon
3. Follow the on screen instructions.

The book's website:
<http://www.library.utoronto.ca/medicine/ebm/>

The website for this book attacks the third of its shortcomings. It will *update its contents, resource lists, and tables* whenever, and as soon as, new evidence, strategies, and tactics come to light. In addition it will *provide links to other evidence-based websites and resources*, including those that provide descriptions and schedules for workshops on how to practice and teach EBM. Moreover, it will provide *a means for contacting the authors* to give us feedback, point out errors in the text, and make suggestions for subsequent editions.

Icons

This icon highlights teaching methods described in the text.

This icon indicates that there is a link between the text and the coloured cards to be found in the cover pocket.

Contents

Preface   ix

Acknowledgements   xiii

Introduction   1

Asking answerable clinical questions   13

How to find current best evidence
and have current best evidence find us   29

Diagnosis and screening   67

Prognosis   95

Therapy   105

Harm   155

Guidelines   169

Teaching Methods   183

Evaluation   219

Appendix 1: Confidence Intervals   233

Appendix 2: Glossary   245

Index   253

The CD

Practicing and Teaching Evidence-Based Health Care in Other Clinical Disciplines

Alternative Medicine

Child Health

Critical Care Medicine

Developing Countries

Gastroenterology and Hepatology

General Practice

Geriatric Medicine

Mental Health

Neonatal Medicine

Nursing

Occupational Therapy

Physiotherapy

Purchasing

Surgery

Evidence-Based Resources

Journals

Books

Computer Software

Websites

The book's website

http://www.library.utoronto.ca/medicine/ebm/search.htm

Preface

This book is for clinicians at any stage of their training or career who want to learn how to practice and teach evidence-based medicine. Written for the busy practitioner, it is short, lean, and highly practical. Those who want, and have time for, more detailed discussions of the theoretical and methodological bases for the tactics described here should consult one of the longer textbooks on clinical epidemiology.*

But this book differs from the others not only in its brevity. Its shift in focus (from theory and explanation to tactics and clinical applications) reflects our growing ability to transform critical appraisals of evidence into direct clinical action. This shift in focus also grows from the continuing clinical experiences of its authors. For Dave Sackett, the ideas behind this book have received a boost every time he's gone through postgraduate training in internal medicine. When his first training (in the US in the 1960s, including clinical and bench research in nephrology) was interrupted by the Cuban missile crisis and 2 years on active duty performing surveys of cardiovascular disease, it dawned on him that epidemiology and biostatistics could be made as relevant to clinical medicine as his research into the tubular transport of amino acids. Twenty years later, after starting a new sort of department (Clinical Epidemiology & Biostatistics) at a new sort of medical school (Canada's McMaster University), he "retreaded" for 2 years as a resident/registrar in general medicine and confirmed (at least in his own mind!) that some basic elements of epidemiology and biostatistics could not only help him critically appraise clinical evidence for its validity and potential usefulness, but also begin to translate that critical appraisal into

---

* The ones we consult are the third edition of *Clinical Epidemiology, The Essentials* (Fletcher RH, Fletcher SW, Wagner EH; Baltimore: Williams & Wilkins, 1996); *Clinical Epidemiology and Biostatistics* (Kramer MS; Berlin: Springer-Verlag, 1988); and our own second edition of *Clinical Epidemiology: A Basic Science for Clinical Medicine* (Sackett DL, Haynes RB, Guyatt GH, Tugwell P; Boston: Little Brown, 1991).

clinical action. By his third stint as a postgraduate trainee, a 1-day posting as a Senior Registrar in Oxford in 1995 (required for colonials with aspirations to NHS consultancy), some wonderful colleagues had helped him develop and describe the applied arm of this basic science to the point where it could be integrated with individual clinical expertise to make individual clinical decisions. During his final 5 years of clinical practice at the John Radcliffe Hospital, his brilliant students and house staff and his wonderfully warm patients helped him confirm that we can practice real EBM in real time on a busy (200+ admissions per month) in-patient service.

As a medical student on a general medicine ward, Sharon Straus was challenged by a senior resident to provide evidence to support her management plans for each patient she admitted. This was so much more exciting than some previous rotations, where the management plan was learned by rote and was based on whatever the current consultant favored. Subsequently, she was fortunate to train in internal medicine at a hospital where the director of medicine was a proponent of clinical epidemiology and actively encouraged evidence-based practice. With encouragement from him, she undertook postgraduate training in clinical epidemiology and this further stimulated her interest in EBM, leading to a fellowship with Dave Sackett in Oxford. An initial 1-year stay in Oxford was extended to an incredible 3-year experience and her enthusiasm for practicing and teaching EBM continued to grow. She hopes that this has led to improved patient care and to more fun and challenge for her medical students.

For Scott Richardson, the ideas for this book began coming together slowly, like the stillness in the shimmering heat of a desert high noon. A flicker of movement started when, as a beginning clinical clerk, he was told by a teacher to read an article to decide what to do for his patient. Perhaps reflecting his teacher's disclaimer that "of course, nobody really does that!" the ideas crept slowly through Scott's residency as he tried to use the literature but found few tools to help him do so. The ideas began to shuffle and shake when he came across the notions of clinical epidemiology and critical appraisal, and grew into a recognizable dance as he used them in his practice and teaching of students and postgraduates at the University of Rochester. The dance of ideas was set to music when Scott began working with others in evidence-based medicine (including these co-authors), fashioning those earlier ideas into clinician-friendly tools for everyday use. Now in San Antonio, this fiesta of ideas is in full swing, as Scott has joined a team with the mission of advancing the science of getting research into practice. The bounce and swing to the beat are from the heap big fun Scott has had learning from and teaching with a large number of EBM colleagues around the world, all working to improve the care of patients by making better use of the best available evidence.

In 1992, Muir Gray introduced William Rosenberg to clinical epidemiology and encouraged him to visit McMaster University. What he learnt there seemed to provide many solutions to the problems he had experienced in trying to articulate clinical questions, integrate learning and teaching with patient care and make this whole process explicit. On his return from Canada, along with colleagues in Oxford, he started to run training sessions in EBM for registrars and clinical students. A year later David Sackett arrived in Oxford and the Centre for Evidence-Based Medicine was established. Since then, first in Oxford and now in Southampton, EBM has come to underpin his learning, practice and teaching. He has enjoyed the pleasure and inspiration of developing EBM with colleagues from many different backgrounds through numerous teaching sessions across the UK and continental Europe and through participation in workshops in Oxford, Cornwall and Wales. He continues to attempt to investigate the effectiveness of EBM and relishes the challenge of trying to practice and teach clinical medicine based on evidence.

Brian Haynes started worrying about the relationship between evidence and clinical practice during his second year of medical school when a psychiatrist gave a lecture on Freud's theories. When asked, "What's the evidence that Freud's theories were correct?", the psychiatrist admitted that there wasn't any good evidence, and that he didn't believe the theories, but he had been asked by the head of the department "to give the talk". This eventually led him to a career combining clinical practice with research in clinical epidemiology to "get the evidence" – only to find that the evidence being generated by medical researchers around the world wasn't getting to practitioners and patients in a timely and dependable way. Sabbaticals permitted a career shift into medical informatics to look into how knowledge is disseminated and applied, and how practitioners and patients can use and benefit from "current best evidence". This led to the development of several evidence-based information resources including *ACP Journal Club, Evidence-Based Medicine, Evidence-Based Nursing, Evidence-Based Mental Health*, and *Best Evidence*, to make it easier for practitioners to get at the best current evidence.

A note about our choice of words: we'll talk about "our" patients throughout this book, not to imply any possession or control of them by us, but to signify that we have taken on an obligation and responsibility to care for and serve each of them.

We're sure that this book contains several errors – we just don't know (yet!) what and where they are. When you find them, please jump on our website and tell us about them. In return, we'll credit your eagle eyes as we correct the next printing.

For the contents of this book to benefit your patients, you readers have to add four ingredients. First, you have to add a mastery of the clinical skills of patient-interviewing, history-taking, and physical examination, without which you can neither begin the process of EBM (by generating diagnostic hypotheses) nor end it (by integrating valid, important evidence with your patient's values and expectations). Second, you must add the practice of continuous, lifelong, self-directed learning, without which you will rapidly become dangerously out of date. Third, you should maintain the humility without which you will become immune both to self-improvement and to advances in medicine. Finally, we implore you to add the enthusiasm and irreverence to the endeavor without which you will miss the fun that accompanies the application of these ideas!

The CD

Practicing and Teaching Evidence-Based Health Care in Other Clinical Disciplines

Alternative Medicine

Child Health

Critical Care Medicine

Developing Countries

Gastroenterology and Hepatology

General Practice

Geriatric Medicine

Mental Health

Neonatal Medicine

Nursing

Occupational Therapy

Physiotherapy

Purchasing

Surgery

Evidence-Based Resources

Journals

Books

Computer Software

Websites

The book's website

http://www.library.utoronto.ca/medicine/ebm/

The number of individuals who gave wonderfully warm and candid feedback on the first edition of the book now exceeds 1000, and we give special thanks to Kathleen McCloskey, S Satya-Murti, Jens Tuerp and Takahiro Okamoto, who pointed out typos that we were able to correct in later printings. Colleagues who offered important suggestions for this edition include Gloria Adams, Chris Ball, Andrew Booth, Antonino Cartabellotta, Iain Chalmers, Martin Dawes, Paul Glasziou, Jeremy Grimshaw, Bruce Guthrie, Mark Loveland, Barry Markovitz, Thomas McGinn, Henry McQuay, Andrew Moore, Doug Morgan, Takahiro Okamoto, Bob Phillips, Francisco Pozo, Nick Shenker, Vasiliy Vlassov, William Woodhouse, Rex Force, and their Family Practice Residents at Idaho State University, plus the 70 medical students who held their own Conferences on Critical Appraisal for Medical Students at Oxford (OCCAMS) and Manchester (MACCAMS) and the more than 2000 participants at the UK Consortium Workshops on How to Practice and Teach EBM held in the UK and on the continent.

We're still seeking better ways of explaining these ideas and their clinical application, and will acknowledge readers' suggestions in subsequent editions of this book. In the meanwhile, we take cheerful responsibility for the parts of the current edition that are still fuzzy, wrong, or boring.

Introduction

WHAT IS EBM?

Evidence-based medicine (EBM) is the integration of best research evidence with clinical expertise and patient values.

- By *best research evidence* we mean clinically relevant research, often from the basic sciences of medicine, but especially from patient-centered clinical research into the accuracy and precision of diagnostic tests (including the clinical examination), the power of prognostic markers, and the efficacy and safety of therapeutic, rehabilitative, and preventive regimens. New evidence from clinical research both invalidates previously accepted diagnostic tests and treatments and replaces them with new ones that are more powerful, more accurate, more efficacious, and safer.

- By *clinical expertise* we mean the ability to use our clinical skills and past experience to rapidly identify each patient's unique health state and diagnosis, their individual risks and benefits of potential interventions, and their personal values and expectations.

- By *patient values* we mean the unique preferences, concerns and expectations each patient brings to a clinical encounter and which must be integrated into clinical decisions if they are to serve the patient.

When these three elements are integrated, clinicians and patients form a diagnostic and therapeutic alliance which optimizes clinical outcomes and quality of life.

WHY THE SUDDEN INTEREST IN EBM?

These ideas have been around for a long time. The authors of this book identify with their expression in post-revolutionary Paris (when clinicians like Pierre Louis rejected the pronouncements of authorities* and sought the truth in systematic observation of patients), and a colleague has nominated a much earlier origin in ancient Chinese medicine.† In the current era, they were consolidated and named EBM in 1992 by a group led by Gordon Guyatt at McMaster University in Canada.[1] Since then, the number of articles about evidence-based practice has grown exponentially (from one publication in 1992 to about 1000 in 1998) and international interest has led to the development of six evidence-based journals (published in up to six languages) that summarize the most relevant studies for clinical practice and have a combined worldwide circulation of over 175 000.

The subsequent rapid spread of EBM has arisen from four realizations and is made possible by five recent developments. The realizations, attested to by ever-increasing numbers of clinicians, are:

1. our daily need for valid information about diagnosis, prognosis, therapy and prevention (up to five times per in-patient[2] and twice for every three outpatients[3])

2. the inadequacy of traditional sources for this information because they are out of date (textbooks[4]), frequently wrong (experts[5]), ineffective (didactic continuing medical education[6]) or too overwhelming in their volume and too variable in their validity for practical clinical use (medical journals[7])

3. the disparity between our diagnostic skills and clinical judgement, which increase with experience, and our up-to-date knowledge[8] and clinical performance,[9] which decline

4. our inability to afford more than a few seconds per patient for finding and assimilating this evidence,[10] or to set aside more than half an hour per week for general reading and study.[11]

---

* For us, Louis's most dramatic rejection was the authoritarian pronouncement that venesection was good for cholera!

† During the reign of Emperor Qianlong, the method of "kaozheng" ("practicing evidential research") was used to interpret ancient Confucian texts (Woodhouse, personal communication, 1998).

Until recently, these problems were insurmountable for full-time clinicians. However, five developments have permitted us to turn this state of affairs around:

1. the development of strategies for efficiently tracking down and appraising evidence (for its validity and relevance)[12]

2. the creation of systematic reviews and concise summaries of the effects of health care (epitomized by the Cochrane Collaboration[13])

3. the creation of evidence-based journals of secondary publication (that publish the 2% of clinical articles that are both valid and of immediate clinical use‡)

4. the creation of information systems for bringing the foregoing to us in seconds[10]

5. the identification and application of effective strategies for lifelong learning and for improving our clinical performance.[14]

This book is devoted to describing these innovations, demonstrating their application to clinical problems, and showing how they can be learned and practiced by clinicians who have just 30 minutes per week to devote to their continuing professional development.

HOW DO WE ACTUALLY PRACTICE EBM?

The full-blown practice of EBM comprises five steps, and this book takes them up in turn:

- *Step 1* – converting the need for information (about prevention, diagnosis, prognosis, therapy, causation, etc.) into an answerable question (Ch. 1)

- *Step 2* – tracking down the best evidence with which to answer that question (Ch. 2)

---

‡ At the time of writing, this list comprised (in order of first publication) *ACP Journal Club, Evidence-Based Medicine*, Journal of *Evidence-Based Health Care, Evidence-Based Cardiovascular Medicine, Evidence-Based Mental Health, Evidence-Based Nursing*, and a growing number of "best-evidence" departments in existing journals.

- *Step 3* – critically appraising that evidence for its validity (closeness to the truth), impact (size of the effect), and applicability (usefulness in our clinical practice) (the first halves of Chs 3 – 7)

- *Step 4* – integrating the critical appraisal with our clinical expertise and with our patient's unique biology, values and circumstances (the second halves of Chs 3 – 7)

- *Step 5* – evaluating our effectiveness and efficiency in executing steps 1 – 4 and seeking ways to improve them both for next time (Ch. 9).

When we examine our practice and that of our colleagues and trainees in this five-step fashion, we can identify three different "modes" or "styles" of practice. All of them involve the integration of evidence (from whatever source) with our patient's unique biology, values and circumstances of step 4, but they vary in the execution of the other steps. For the conditions we encounter every day (e.g. unstable angina and venous thromboembolism) we need to be "up to the minute" and very sure about what we are doing. Accordingly, we invest the time and effort necessary to carry out both steps 2 (searching) and 3 (critically appraising), and operate in the "appraising" mode; all the chapters in this book are relevant to the "appraising" mode.

For the conditions we encounter less often (e.g. temporal arteritis, aspirin poisoning), we conserve our time by seeking out critical appraisals already performed by others who describe (and stick to!) explicit criteria for deciding what evidence they selected and how they decided whether it was valid. That is, we leave out the time-consuming step 3 (critically appraising) and carry out just step 2 (searching) but restrict the latter to sources that have already undergone rigorous critical appraisal (*Cochrane Reviews*, *Best Evidence*, and the like[§]). Only the third portions ("Can I apply this valid, important evidence to my patient?") of Chapters 3 – 7

[§] Contains a list of pre-appraised resources, and examples appear on the accompanying CD. This list is kept up to date on the book's website: http://www.library.utoronto.ca/medicine/ebm/

are strictly relevant here, and the growing database of pre-appraised resources is making this "searching" mode more and more feasible for busy clinicians. The reassuring thing about practicing in either the "appraising" or "searching" modes is that we can be pretty sure that we are providing "evidence-based care" to our patients.

This reassurance is lacking from the third mode of practice. For the problems we're likely to encounter very infrequently (the last example from the Sackett/Straus service was a man who developed bad pneumonia while trying to reject his heart–lung transplant), we "blindly" seek, accept and apply the recommendations we receive from authorities in the relevant branch of medicine. This "replicating" mode also characterizes the practice of medical students and clinical trainees when they haven't yet been granted independence and have to carry out the orders of their consultants. The trouble with the "replicating" mode is that it is "blind" to whether the advice received from the experts is authoritative (evidence-based, resulting from their operating in the "appraising" mode) or merely authoritarian (opinion-based, resulting from pride and prejudice). Sometimes we can gain clues about the validity of our expert source (Do they cite references? Are they a member of the Cochrane Collaboration?). If we tracked the care we give when operating in the "replicating" mode into the literature and critically appraised it, we would find that some of it was effective, some useless, and some harmful. But in the "replicating" mode we'll never be sure which.

CAN CLINICIANS ACTUALLY PRACTICE EBM?

First of all, do full-time clinicians really recognize working in these modes? It appears so. In a survey of UK GPs (in which responders were more likely to hold MRCP certification), the great majority reported practicing at least part of their time in the "searching" mode, using evidence-based summaries generated by others (72%) and evidence-based practice guidelines or protocols (84%).[15] On the other hand, far fewer claimed to understand (and to be able to explain) the "appraising" tools of NNTs (35%) and confidence intervals (20%). Finally only 5% believed that "learning the skills of evidence-based medicine" (all five steps) was the most appropriate method for "moving from opinion-based medicine to evidence-based medicine".**

Second, even if they recognize these modes, can they actually get at the evidence quickly enough to consider it on a busy clinical service? Again, it appears so, but examples are few. When a busy (180+ admissions per month) in-patient medical service brought electronic summaries of evidence previously appraised either by team members ("CATs"††) or by the summary journals‡‡ to working rounds, it was documented that, on average, the former could be accessed in 10 seconds and the latter in 25.[10] Moreover, when assessed from the viewpoint of the most junior member of the team caring for the patient, this evidence changed 25% of their diagnostic and treatment suggestions and added to a further 23% of them.

Third, even if they can get at it, can clinicians actually provide evidence-based care to their patients? Again, it appears so from audits carried out on clinical services that attempt to operate in the searching and appraising modes. The first of these examined the evidence base for the primary interventions applied to the primary diagnoses of consecutive patients on an in-patient medical service and documented that 82% of them were evidence-based (53% based on randomized trials or systematic reviews of randomized trials and 29% based on convincing non-experimental evidence).[16] Similar results have been obtained from audits of psychiatric,[17] surgical,[18] pediatric[19] and general[20] practice.

DOES PROVIDING EVIDENCE-BASED CARE IMPROVE OUTCOMES FOR PATIENTS?

No such evidence is available from randomized trials because no investigative team or research granting agency has yet overcome the problems of sample size, contamination,

---

** As it happens, this latter result is surprisingly close to a 1981 guestimate by the authors of the McMaster University readers guides that only 6% of clinicians would be likely to master and use critical appraisal skills (Sackett DL, Haynes RB, Tugwell P, Neufeld VR, personal communication, 1999.)

†† CATs, or "critically appraised topics", are discussed on page 87.

‡‡ *Best Evidence*, described on page 32. "

blinding, and long-term follow-up which such a trial requires. Moreover, there are ethical concerns with such a trial: is withholding access to evidence from the control clinicians ethical? On the other hand, population-based "outcomes research" has repeatedly documented that those patients who do receive evidence-based therapies have better outcomes than those who don't. For positive examples, myocardial infarction survivors prescribed aspirin or beta-blockers have lower mortality rates than those who aren't prescribed these drugs,[21,22] and where clinicians use more warfarin and stroke unit referrals, stroke mortality declines by >20%.[23] For a negative example, patients undergoing carotid surgery despite failing to meet evidence-based operative criteria, when compared with operated patients who meet those criteria, are more than three times as likely to suffer major stroke or death in the next month.[24]

WHAT ARE THE LIMITATIONS OF EBM?

The examination of the concepts and practice of EBM by clinicians and academics has led to negative as well as positive reactions. The ensuing discussion and debate has reminded us of three limitations that are universal to science (whether basic or applied) and medicine – the shortage of coherent, consistent scientific evidence; difficulties in applying any evidence to the care of individual patients; barriers to any practice of high-quality medicine. The debate has also identified three limitations that are unique to the practice of EBM.[25,26] First, the need to develop new skills in searching and critical appraisal can be daunting, although (as we pointed out above) evidence-based care can still be applied if only the former has been mastered and directed toward pre-appraised resources. Second, busy clinicians have limited time to master and apply these new skills, and the resources required for instant access to evidence are often woefully inadequate in clinical settings. Finally, evidence that EBM "works" has been late and slow to come.

On the other hand, the ensuing discussion and debate has clarified some "pseudo-limitations" that arise from misunderstandings of the definition of EBM. An examination of the definition and steps of EBM quickly dismisses the criticisms that it denigrates clinical expertise, is limited to clinical research, ignores patients' values and preferences, or promotes a cookbook approach to medicine. Moreover, it is not an effective cost-cutting tool, since providing evidence-based care directed toward maximizing patients' quality of life often increases the costs of their care and raises the ire of health economists.[27] In addition, the self-reported employment of the "searching" mode by a great majority of front-line GPs dispels the contention that EBM is an ivory tower concept. Finally, we hope that the rest of this book will put to rest the concern that EBM leads to therapeutic nihilism in the absence of randomized trial evidence.

WHAT ARE THE OTHER USES OF EBM?

Although the prime focus of this book is how to master and use EBM in making decisions around the problems of individual patients, several other uses have been recognized:

- It reinforces the need for, and mastery of, the clinical and communication skills that are required to gather and critically appraise patients' stories, symptoms, and signs and to identify and incorporate their values and expectations into therapeutic alliances.

- It fosters generic skills for use in finding, appraising and implementing evidence from the basic sciences and from other applied sciences.

- It provides an effective, efficient framework for postgraduate education and self-directed, lifelong learning; when coupled with "virtual libraries" and distance learning programs, it supplies a model of worldwide applicability.

- Although not its primary aim, by identifying the questions for which no satisfactory evidence exists it generates a supremely pragmatic agenda for applied health research (that is formally recognized by groups such as the UK NHS R&D Programme).

- As shown in the CD that accompanies this book, it provides a common language for use by the multidisciplinary teams whose effective collaboration is essential if patients are to benefit from new knowledge.

HOW IS THIS PACKAGE (THE BOOK, THE ACCOMPANYING CD, AND THE ASSOCIATED WEBSITE) ORGANIZED?

The overall package is designed to help practitioners from any health care discipline learn how to practice evidence-based health care. Thus, although the book is written within the narrow perspective of internal medicine, the CD provides clinical scenarios, questions, searches, critical appraisals, and evidence summaries from 14 other disciplines,§§ permitting readers to apply the strategies and tactics of evidence-based practice to any health discipline.

The book's organization begins with the first two steps of practicing EBM, so Chapter 1 describes how to form clinical questions so that they can be answered, and Chapter 2 how to search for the best research evidence. Based on readers' feedback on our first edition, the next sections of the book on how to critically appraise the evidence unearthed by steps 1 and 2 have been reorganized on the basis of the clinical problem to be solved – "diagnosis and screening" in Chapter 3, "prognosis" in Chapter 4, "therapy" in Chapter 5, and "harm" in Chapter 6. Those of you who want to practice full-blown EBM are encouraged to struggle through the lot (the order of Chs 3–6 dictated by the order in which your clinical practice generates questions for you and your patients). On the other hand, those of you who want to start by (or limit yourselves to) mastering the "evidence-based searching" mode can attack Chapters 1 and 2 with a major focus on pre-appraised resources and then take on just the third portions ("Can I apply this valid, important evidence to my patient?") of Chapters 3–6.

Guidelines got their own chapter (Ch. 7), not only because they often apply to both diagnosis and therapy, but also because readers are often invited to generate as well as use them. And because this book is also intended to help its readers learn how to teach EBM, we've included tips about teaching throughout it and added full chapters on teaching (Ch. 8) and evaluation (Ch. 9).

§§ For a complete listing, see the Table of Contents.

The chapters and appendices that comprise this book constitute a traditional way of presenting our ideas about EBM. Although it may suffice for some of you, we think our book suffers from three major shortcomings: First, its clinical examples are constricted by the narrow clinical perspective of the general physicians who wrote it; readers from other branches of medicine, and especially from other health professions, face the frustrating (but hopefully fulfilling) task of transposing the lessons to their own patients and settings. Second, the descriptions of evidence sources are restricted by the limits of print space (and the size of your pockets!). Finally, this book is stuck in amber, and parts of it (written in early 1999) will be out of date by the time it appears in print (in late 1999).

We've decided to try to overcome these deficiencies by employing some of the same innovations in information packaging (the accompanying CD) and communication (the book's website) that have made the modern practice of EBM possible.

The accompanying compact disk

The CD tucked inside the cover of this book attacks the first and second of the book's shortcomings. First, it contains *clinical examples, critical appraisals, and background papers from 14 other health disciplines*. As a result, health professionals from these other disciplines can substitute them for the examples and appraisals in this book and much more easily integrate its message into their own clinical practice. Second, it contains *extended descriptions (including sample web pages) of several current evidence sources* regularly consulted by the authors of this book.

The book's website: <http://www.library.utoronto.ca/medicine/ebm/>

The website for this book attacks the third of its shortcomings. It will *update its contents, resource lists, and tables* whenever, and as soon as, new evidence, strategies, and tactics come to light. In addition, it will *provide links to other evidence-based websites and resources*, including those that provide descriptions and schedules for workshops in how to practice and teach EBM. Moreover, it will *provide a means for contacting the authors* to give us feedback, point out errors in the text, and make suggestions for subsequent editions.

References

1   Evidence-Based Medicine Working Group. Evidence-based medicine. A new approach to teaching the practice of medicine. JAMA 1992; 268: 2420–5.

2   Osheroff J A, Forsythe D E, Buchanan B G, Bankowitz R A, Blumenfeld B H, Miller R A. Physicians' information needs: analysis of questions posed during clinical teaching. Ann Intern Med 1991; 114: 576–81.

3   Covell D G, Uman G C, Manning P R. Information needs in office practice: are they being met? Ann Intern Med 1985; 103: 596–9.

4   Antman E M, Lau J, Kupelnick B, Mosteller F, Chalmers T C. A comparison of results of meta-analyses of randomised control trials and recommendations of clinical experts. JAMA 1992; 268: 240–8.

5   Oxman A, Guyatt G H. The science of reviewing research. Ann NY Acad Sci 1993; 703: 125–34.

6   Davis D A, Thomson M A, Oxman A D, Haynes R B. Changing physician performance: a systematic review of the effect of continuing medical education strategies. JAMA 1997; 274: 700–5.

7   Haynes R B. Where's the meat in clinical journals [editorial]? ACP Journal Club 1993; 119: A-22–3.

8   Evans C E, Haynes R B, Birkett N J et al. Does a mailed continuing education program improve clinician performance? Results of a randomised trial in antihypertensive care. JAMA 1986; 255: 501–4.

9   Sackett D L, Haynes R B, Taylor D W, Gibson E S, Roberts R S, Johnson A L. Clinical determinants of the decision to treat primary hypertension. Clinical Research 1977; 24: 648.

10 Sackett D L, Straus S E. Finding and applying evidence during clinical rounds: the "evidence cart". JAMA 1998; 280: 1336–8.

11 Sackett D L. Using evidence-based medicine to help physicians keep up-to-date. Serials 1997; 9: 178–81.

12 Sackett D L, Richardson W S, Rosenberg W, Haynes R B. Evidence-based medicine: how to practice and teach EBM. Churchill Livingstone, London, 1997. (Published in English, Spanish, Italian, and Japanese.)

13 The Cochrane Library, Issue 2. Update Software, Oxford, 1999.

14 Cochrane Effective Practice and Organisation of Care Group. The Cochrane Library, Issue 2. Update Software, Oxford, 1999.

15 McColl A, Smith H, White P, Field J. General practitioners' perceptions of the route to evidence based medicine: a questionnaire survey. BMJ 1998; 316: 361–5.

16 Ellis J, Mulligan I, Rowe J, Sackett D L. Inpatient general medicine is evidence based. Lancet 1995; 346: 407–10. *This whole series of studies are summarised and updated by Andrew Booth on his excellent website: <http://www.shef.ac.uk/~scharr/ir/percent.html>*

17 Geddes J R, Game D, Jenkins N E, Peterson L A, Pottinger G R, Sackett D L. In-patient psychiatric care is evidence-based. Proceedings of the Royal College of Psychiatrists Winter Meeting, Stratford, UK, January 23–25, 1996.

18 Howes N, Chagla L, Thorpe M, McCulloch P. Surgical practice is evidence based. Br J Surg 1997; 84: 1220–3.

19 Kenny S E, Shankar K R, Rintala R, Lamont G L, Lloyd D A. Evidence-based surgery: interventions in a regional paediatric surgical unit. Arch Dis Child 1997; 76: 50–3.

20 Gill P, Dowell A C, Neal R D, Smith N, Heywood P, Wilson A E. Evidence based general practice: a retrospective study of interventions in one training practice. BMJ 1996; 312: 819–21.

21 Krumholz H M, Radford M J, Ellerbeck E F et al. Aspirin for secondary prevention after acute myocardial infarction in the elderly: prescribed use and outcomes. Ann Intern Med 1996; 124: 292–8.

22 Krumholz H M, Radford M J, Wang Y, Chen J, Heiat A, Marciniak T A. National use and effectiveness of beta-blockers for the treatment of elderly patients after acute myocardial infarction. National Cooperative Cardiovascular Project. JAMA 1998; 280: 623–9.

23 Mitchell J B, Ballard D J, Whisnant J P, Ammering C J, Samsa G P, Matchar D B. What role do neurologists play in determining the costs and outcomes of stroke patients? Stroke 1996; 27: 1937–43.

24 Wong J H, Findlay J M, Suarez-Almazor M E. Regional performance of carotid endarterectomy appropriateness, outcomes and risk factors for complications. Stroke 1997; 28: 891–8.

25 Sackett D L, Rosenberg W M C, Gray J A M, Haynes R B, Richardson W S. Evidence based medicine: what it is and what it isn't. BMJ 1996; 312: 71–2.

26 Straus S E, McAlister F A. The limitations of evidence-based medicine. In press.

27 Maynard A. Evidence-based medicine: an incomplete method for informing treatment choices. Lancet 1997; 349: 126–8.

As we stated in the Introduction, almost every time we see a patient we will need new information about some element of their diagnosis, prognosis or management. Sometimes what we need will be self-evident and the necessary information will be at our fingertips. At other times our information needs will not be so obvious, and the necessary information will be in the form of external evidence we will have to track down. For many clinicians, the efforts required to both ask questions and track down answers are so formidable that, when coupled with our very limited time for reading and keeping up to date, most of our information needs never get met.

In this book we'll do our best to provide powerful and efficient ways to fill some of those information needs, and in this chapter we will describe a strategy for formulating answerable clinical questions as the first step in practicing EBM. In our experience, this is the hardest step that many people face in finding best current evidence to address clinical problems. Because EBM begins and ends with patients, we will use a patient encounter to remind us how clinical questions arise and to show how they can be used to initiate evidence-based learning. We will also introduce some teaching tactics that can help us coach others to develop their questioning skills. If you think you already know how to ask answerable questions (although you may want to make sure by trying the example!), skip the early portions of this chapter and go straight to the section on how to teach the asking of answerable clinical questions.

An example

Suppose you've just accepted the invitation of one of your colleagues to join her in-patient clinical team on rounds. The team has finished admitting a patient and they are ready to present to your colleague. The patient is a 77-year-old man admitted for dyspnea and fever. He fell ill 4 days ago with low-grade fever, chills, myalgias, rhinorrhoea and a non-productive cough. One day ago he developed dyspnea on exertion, purulent sputum, lateral chest wall pain with inspiration and a shaking chill. His general health is fairly good; he has had essential hypertension for 12 years, well controlled on diuretic therapy. He has not smoked. He is independent in his activities of daily living. He lives alone now, after his wife died 3 years ago. On examination, his respiratory rate is 28, his heart rate is 108 and his temperature is 39.2°C. He may have subtle cyanosis. His chest expands symmetrically, he has no prolongation of expiration and no wheezing. There is bronchophony and egophony in the left lower posterior lung field. Initial blood tests show leukocytosis and hyponatremia. The team suspects acute community-acquired pneumonia with hypoxemia, and plans chest radiographs, sputum studies, supplemental oxygen and antimicrobial therapy.

Your consultant colleague then asks her team what questions they have about this case: what important pieces of medical knowledge they'd like to have in order to provide better care for this patient. What do you suppose these might be? What questions occur to you about this patient? Write the first three of your questions in the boxes below:

1.

2.

3.

The first three questions asked by the team's students were:

(a) What microbial organisms can cause community-acquired pneumonia?

(b) How does pneumonia cause egophony?

(c) What do patients mean by calling pneumonia "the old man's friend"?

What do you make of them?

TYPES OF QUESTIONS

Notice that the students' questions (above) ask for general or "background" knowledge about pneumonia, the disorder that presumably explains much of this patient's acute illness. When well formulated, such "background" questions usually have two components (see Table 1.1):

Table 1.1 Well-built clinical questions

"Background" questions
- Ask for general knowledge about a disorder
- Have two essential components:
  1. A question root (who, what, where, when, how, why) with a verb
  2. A disorder, or an aspect of a disorder

Examples:

"What causes babesiosis?"
"When do complications of acute pancreatitis usually occur?"

"Foreground" questions
- Ask for specific knowledge about managing patients with a disorder
- Have four (or three) essential components:
  1. Patient and/or problem
  2. Intervention
  3. Comparison intervention (if relevant)
  4. Clinical outcomes

Example:

"In older patients with heart failure from isolated diastolic dysfunction, does adding digoxin to standard diuretic and ACE inhibitor treatment yield enough reduction in morbidity and/or mortality to be worth its adverse effects?"

1. a question root with a verb (e.g. "what causes...?" or "how does...?")

2. some aspect of the disorder itself (e.g. cyanosis, hypoxemia).

Note also that "background" questions can cover the full range of biologic, psychological or sociologic aspects of human health and illness.

The team's house officers asked several questions, too, including:

(a) In patients with suspected pneumonia, are any clinical findings sufficiently powerful to confirm or exclude pneumonia all by themselves, or is a chest radiograph necessary for the diagnosis?

(b) In patients with community-acquired pneumonia, is the probability of *Legionella* infection sufficiently high to warrant considering covering this organism with the initial antibiotic choice?

(c) In patients with community-acquired pneumonia, do clinical features predict outcome well enough that "low risk" patients can be treated safely at home?

Notice that these questions ask for specific knowledge about how to diagnose, "prognose", and treat patients with pneumonia, which might be called "foreground" knowledge. When well built, such "foreground" questions usually have four components (see Table 1.1):

1. The patient and/or problem of interest

2. The main intervention (defined very broadly, including an exposure, a diagnostic test, a prognostic factor, a treatment, a patient perception, and so forth)

3. Comparison intervention(s), if relevant

4. The clinical outcome(s) of interest.

Just like "background" questions, "foreground" questions can cover a wide range of biologic, psychological and sociologic aspects of caring for sick persons.

Go back to the three questions you wrote down about our patient. Are they "background" or "foreground" questions? Do your "background" questions specify the two components (root with verb and condition), and do your "foreground" questions contain three or four components (patient/problem, intervention, comparison, and outcome)? If not, try rewriting them to include these components, and consider whether these revised questions are clearer.

As clinicians, we all have needs for both "background" and "foreground" knowledge, in proportions that vary over time and that depend primarily on our experience with the particular disorder at hand (see Fig. 1.1). When our experience with the condition is limited, at point "A" (like a beginning student), the majority of our questions (designated in the figure by the vertical dimension) might be about "background" knowledge. As we grow in clinical experience and responsibility, such as at point "B" (like a house officer), we'll have increasing proportions of questions about the "foreground" of managing patients. Further experience with the condition puts us at point "C", where most of our questions will be "foreground". Notice the diagonal line is placed to show that we're never too green to learn "foreground" knowledge, nor too experienced to outlive the need for "background" knowledge.

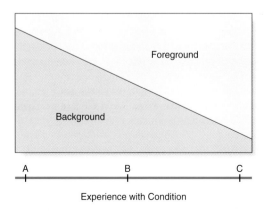

Figure 1.1 Background and foreground questions.

Clinical practice demands that we use large amounts of both "background" and "foreground" knowledge. If a clinical situation calls for knowledge that we already possess, we experience the reinforcing mental and emotional responses that have been called "cognitive resonance" and can make rapid decisions. But if our patient's illness calls for knowledge that we don't possess, we experience mental and emotional responses termed "cognitive dissonance", and this can be a powerful motivator. Sometimes it motivates us to develop maladaptive reactions to cognitive dissonance, either by trying to hide our knowledge deficit from ourselves, or by overreacting emotionally with excessive anxiety, guilt or shame. A more positive ("adaptive") response is to recognize our information needs and use our cognitive dissonance to motivate our learning, by turning the "negative space" of knowledge gaps into the "positive space" of well-built questions and finding answers. (There is an even darker side to not knowing that goes by several names, including ignorance, incompetence, obsolescence, and not knowing when we don't know. Since we don't feel any cognitive dissonance with this, the solution is different: regular review of "current best evidence" through processes and publications that are described in Chapter 2 under "Current Awareness.")

WHERE AND HOW CLINICAL QUESTIONS ARISE

As one might expect, over the years we've found that most of our "foreground" questions arise from the central issues involved in caring for patients (see Table 1.2). These groupings are neither jointly exhaustive (other worthwhile questions can be asked), nor mutually exclusive (some questions are "hybrids", asking about, say, both prognosis and therapy). Still, we find it useful to anticipate that many of our questions will arise from common locations on this "map": clinical findings, etiology, differential diagnosis, diagnostic tests, prognosis, therapy, prevention, patient experience and meaning, and self-improvement.

Why bother formulating questions clearly? We know of no controlled trials that demonstrate that doing so leads to better evidence, found faster, and used more wisely in patient care.

Table 1.2 Central issues in clinical work, where clinical questions often arise

1. **Clinical findings**: how to properly gather and interpret findings from the history and physical examination.

2. **Etiology**: how to identify causes for disease (including its iatrogenic forms).

3. **Clinical manifestations of disease**: knowing how often and when a disease causes its clinical manifestations and how to use this knowledge in classifying our patients' illnesses.

4. **Differential diagnosis**: when considering the possible causes of our patient's clinical problem, how to select those that are likely, serious and responsive to treatment.

5. **Diagnostic tests**: how to select and interpret diagnostic tests, in order to confirm or exclude a diagnosis, based on considering their precision, accuracy, acceptability, expense, safety, etc.

6. **Prognosis**: how to estimate our patient's likely clinical course over time and anticipate likely complications of the disorder.

7. **Therapy**: how to select treatments to offer our patients that do more good than harm and that are worth the efforts and costs of using them.

8. **Prevention**: how to reduce the chance of disease by identifying and modifying risk factors and how to diagnose disease early by screening.

9. **Experience and meaning**: how to empathize with our patients' situations, appreciate the meaning they find in the experience and understand how this meaning influences their healing.

10. **Self-improvement**: how to keep up to date, improve my clinical and other skills and run a better, more efficient clinical practice.

All the authors have are our personal case reports that well-formulated questions have helped us in seven ways:

1. They help us focus our scarce learning time on evidence that is directly relevant to our patients' clinical needs.

2. They help us focus our scarce learning time on evidence that directly addresses our particular knowledge needs, or those of our learners.

3. They can suggest high-yield search strategies (see Ch. 2).

4. They suggest the forms that useful answers might take (see Chs 3–6).

5. When sending or receiving a patient in referral, they can help us to communicate clearly with our colleagues.

6. When teaching, they can help our learners to better understand the content of what we teach, while also modeling some adaptive processes for lifelong learning.

7. When we answer our questions, our curiosity is reinforced, our cognitive resonance is restored, and we can become better, faster and happier as clinicians.

PROBLEMS IN POSING ANSWERABLE QUESTIONS

Three problems often impede the posing of answerable questions:

1. *When we're puzzled by a patient but don't know where to start.* When we're stuck but we're not sure where, we scan Table 1.2 and ask ourselves, for each of the ten clinical issues, whether we have any cognitive dissonance or uncertainty. If we can't confidently and quickly answer "No!", we've just found a knowledge gap. We can congratulate ourselves for finding it (rather than hiding it or scolding ourselves), and then turn the "negative space" of the gap into the "positive space" of a question.

2. *When we have trouble articulating the question.* When this happens, we can try saying our questions out loud or writing them down with all their components. If we're stuck, we can use Table 1.2 to locate where we are stuck. Then, we can build our question in two steps, first specifying the central clinical issue and then filling in the components explicitly. For those who are in the habit of writing down clinical questions to answer later, consider dividing the paper into four columns, one for each element of the question, so that questions can be written in quickly as components, rather than as complete sentences.

3. *When we have more questions than time.* This will almost always be the case, so we need to develop a strategy for deciding where to begin. Keep in mind that lifelong learning means learning in many small increments over a long time and attempts to do it all at once are impossible

and therefore bound to frustrate. Factors to consider when deciding which question to answer first include:

- Which question is most important to the patient's well-being?
- Which question is most relevant to our learners' needs?
- Which question is most feasible to answer within the time we have available?
- Which question is most interesting?
- Which question is most likely to recur in our practice?

QUESTIONS OUR PATIENTS WANT ANSWERED

Of course, the questions our patients ask may bear little resemblance to our own. How many times have we assured patients with excruciating abdominal pain that they "only have irritable bowel syndrome" when it had not occurred to them that they might have had cancer, yet still have pain? We need to pause a moment, consider our patient's perspective, and frame a four-part question that will help us assemble the evidence that will help them. This might be initiated by asking them: "What do *you* think is the problem?"; "Have you any thoughts about what treatment you need/want?"; "What alternatives have you heard about/read about/considered?"; "What benefits do you want/need?". Incorporating their responses into our four-part question will ensure patient-centered answers that enhance the quality of our consultations and the care we provide.

Often the questions that we and our patients ask relate to their experience of diseases, diagnostic tests and treatments rather than their test results or health outcomes. Research that explores these issues by asking patients about, or by observing, their experiences of diseases, tests and treatments is called "qualitative research". This type of research seeks to describe and understand patients' feelings, ideas and wider experience rather than measuring objective outcomes. Whilst we regard the integration of qualitative research to be one of the major current challenges in EBM, we readily admit that we are not expert in this field and defer to others. Much of the work in qualitative research has been undertaken by social scientists and particularly by the nursing profession, whose perspective is often that of the patient and whose objective is to obtain greater understanding of their experience of health care. In doing so, they may employ the methodologies of phenomenology, ethnography, grounded theory, "action research" (in which the researcher is an active participant), and "evaluation research" (in which the researcher passively evaluates participants' experiences). The emphasis throughout is on experiences rather than "objective" effects, and these may be ascertained through focus groups, individual interviews, surveys, or participant observation. Some qualitative researchers argue that qualitative research results are unique to the subjects of individual studies and are neither generalizable nor combinable through meta-analysis, whilst others believe that generalizable truths can be extracted from individual experiences.

TEACHING THE ASKING OF ANSWERABLE QUESTIONS

Good questions are the backbone of both practicing and teaching EBM, and patients serve as the starting point for both. Our challenge as teachers is to identify questions that are both patient-based (arising out of the clinical problems of this real patient under the learner's care) and learner-centered (targeting the learning needs of this learner). As we become more skilled at asking questions ourselves, we also become more skilled in teaching others how to do so.

As with other clinical skills, most of us teach question-asking best by example, i.e. by modeling the formation of good clinical questions in front of our learners. By doing this, we can also model admitting that we don't know it all, identifying our own knowledge gaps, and showing our learners adaptive ways of responding to the resulting cognitive dissonance. Once we've modeled asking a few questions, we can stop and describe explicitly what we did, noting each of the elements of good questions, whether "background" or "foreground".

The four main steps in teaching clinical learners how to ask good questions are listed in Table 1.3.

If we are to recognize potential questions in learners' cases, help them select the "best" question to focus on, guide them in building that question well, and assess their question-building

Table 1.3 Key steps in teaching how to ask questions for EBM

1. **Recognize**: how to identify combinations of a patient's needs and a learner's needs that represent opportunities for the learner to build good questions and hone question-asking skills.

2. **Select**: how to select from the recognized opportunities the one (or few) that best fits the needs of the patient and the learner at that clinical moment.

3. **Guide**: how to guide the learner in transforming knowledge gaps into well-built clinical questions.

4. **Assess**: how to assess the learner's performance and skill at asking pertinent, answerable clinical questions for practicing EBM.

performance and skill, we need to be proficient at building questions ourselves. Moreover, we need several attributes of good clinical teaching in general, such as good listening skills, enthusiasm and a willingness to help learners develop to their full potential. It helps to be able to spot signs of our learners' cognitive dissonance, to know when and what they're ready to learn.

Note that teaching question-asking skills can be integrated with any other clinical teaching, right at the bedside or other site of patient care, and it needn't take much additional time. In fact, it'll save learning time in the long run, for our learners will become much more efficient in asking answerable questions, leaving more time for actually learning their answers.

Once we have formulated an important question, how might we keep track of it and follow its progress toward a clinically useful answer? It may be just one of several questions we formulate during a single encounter and it may not be answered for days. One tactic we've used for keeping track, the educational prescription shown in Figure 1.2, helps both teachers and learners in five ways:

1. It specifies the clinical problem that generated the question.

2. It states the question, in all of its key elements.

3. It specifies who is responsible for answering it.

Rx Educational Prescription

Patient's Name	Learner:

3-part Clinical Question

Target Disorder:

Intervention (+/- comparison):

Outcome:

Date and place to be filled:

Presentations will cover:

1. search strategy;
2. search results;
3. the validity of this evidence;
4. the importance of this valid evidence;
5. can this valid, important evidence be applied to your patient;
6. your evaluation of this process.

Figure 1.2 An educational prescription.

4. It reminds everyone of the deadline for answering it (taking into account the urgency of the clinical problem that generated it).

5. Finally, it reminds everyone of the steps of searching, critically appraising and relating the answer back to the patient.

How might we use the educational prescription in clinical teaching? The number of ways is limited only by our imaginations and our opportunities for teaching. As we'll reinforce in Chapter 8 (Teaching methods), educational prescriptions have been incorporated into familiar in-patient teaching settings from work rounds and attending/consultant rounds to morning reports and noon conferences. They have also been used in outpatient teaching settings, such as ambulatory morning report. Some general practitioners we know write them on real prescription blanks and toss them in a tray that they and their colleagues review periodically, taking the recurring themes up as a shared activity throughout the partnership.

Will you and your learners follow through on the educational prescriptions? You might, if you build the writing and "dispensing" of them into your everyday routine. One tactic we use is to make specifying clinical questions an integral part of presenting a new patient to the group. For example, we ask learners on our general medicine in-patient clinical teams, when presenting new patients, to tell us "33 things in 3 minutes" about each admission. As shown in Table 1.4, the final element of their presentations is the specification of an important question to which they need to know the answer and don't. If the answer is vital to the immediate care of the patient, it can be provided at once by another member of the clinical team, perhaps by referring to the record (such as a one-page "CAT")* of the answer generated from posing that same question on an earlier occasion. Most of the time the answer can wait a few hours or days, so the question can serve as the start of an educational prescription.

Finally, we can ask our learners to write educational prescriptions for us. This role reversal can help in four ways:

1. the learners must supervise our question building, thereby honing their skills further

2. the learners see us admitting our own knowledge gaps and practicing what we preach

---

* CATs ("critically appraised topics") are described in detail on p. 87.

Table 1.4 A patient presentation that includes an educational prescription

1. The patient's surname.

2. The patient's age.

3. The patient's gender.

4. When the patient was admitted.

5. The chief complaint(s) that led to admission. For each complaint, mention the following:

    6. Where in the body it is located.

    7. Its quality.

    8. Its quantity, intensity and degree of impairment.

    9. Its chronology: when it began, constant/episodic, progressive.

    10. Its setting: under what circumstances did/does it occur.

    11. Any aggravating or alleviating factors.

    12. Any associated symptoms.

13. Whether a similar complaint had happened previously. If so:

14. How it was investigated.

15. What the patient was told about its cause.

16. How the patient had been treated for it.

17. Pertinent past history of other conditions that are either of prognostic significance or would affect the evaluation or treatment of the chief complaint.

18. And how those other conditions have been treated.

19. Family history, if pertinent to chief complaint or hospital care.

20. Social history, if pertinent to chief complaint or hospital care.

21. Their:

    (a) Ideas (what they think is wrong with them)
    (b) Concerns (about their illness, and other issues)
    (c) Expectations (of what's going to happen to and for them).

22. Their condition on admission:

    (a) acutely and/or chronically ill
    (b) severity
    (c) requesting what sort of help.

23. The pertinent physical findings on admission.

24. The pertinent diagnostic test results.

25. Your concise, one-sentence problem synthesis.

26. What you think the most likely diagnosis is.

27. And the other items in your differential diagnosis.

Table 1.4 (cont'd)

28. Any further diagnostic studies you plan to carry out.

29. Your estimate of the patient's prognosis.

30. Your treatment plans.

31. How you will monitor the treatment.

32. And what you will do if the patient doesn't respond to the treatment.

33. The educational prescription you would like to write for yourself in order to better understand the patient's disorder ("background" knowledge) or how to care for the patient ("foreground" knowledge) in order to become a better clinician.

3. it adds fun to rounds and sustains group morale

4. our learners begin to prepare for their later roles as clinical teachers.

That concludes this chapter on the first step in practicing and teaching EBM: asking answerable clinical questions. Since you and your learners will want to move quickly from asking questions to finding their answers, our next chapter will address this second step in practicing and teaching EBM.

Further reading

Neighbour R. The inner apprentice: an awareness-centered approach to vocational training for general practice. Petroc Press, Newbury (UK), 1996.

Oxman A D, Sackett D L, Guyatt G H, for the Evidence-Based Medicine Working Group. Users' guides to the medical literature: I. How to get started. JAMA 1993; 270: 2093–5.

Richardson W S. Ask, and ye shall retrieve [EBM Note]. Evidence Based Medicine 1998; 3: 100–1.

Richardson W S, Wilson M C, Nishikawa J, Hayward R S A. The well-built clinical question: a key to evidence-based decisions [Editorial]. ACP J Club 1995; 123: A12–3.

Schon D A. Educating the reflective practitioner. Jossey-Bass, San Francisco (US), 1987.

Smith R. What clinical information do doctors need? BMJ 1996; 313: 1062–8.

How to find current best evidence

and how to have current best evidence find us

My students are dismayed when I say to them "Half of what you are taught as medical students will in 10 years have been shown to be wrong. And the trouble is, none of your teachers knows which half."

(Dr Sydney Burwell, Dean of Harvard Medical School)[1]

As highlighted in the Preface, keeping up to date with current best evidence for the care of our patients is challenging. As Dr Burwell's quote from half a century ago indicates, new medical knowledge was evolving quite quickly then. In the past decade, the pace has accelerated because of the maturation of biomedical research (from bench to bedside), and huge new investments in health care research of over US$55bn per year.

One solution for the problem of obsolescence of professional education is "problem-based learning" or "learning by inquiry". That is, when confronted by a clinical question for which we are unsure of the current best answer, we need to develop the habit of looking for the current best answer as efficiently as possible. (Literary critics will point out the redundancy of the term "current best" – we risk their scorn to emphasize that last year's best answer may not be this year's.)

The success of learning by inquiry depends heavily on being able to find the current best evidence to manage pressing clinical problems, a task that can be either quick and highly rewarding or time-consuming and frustrating. Which of these it is depends on several factors that we can control or influence, including which questions we ask, how we ask these questions (see Ch. 1), which information resources we use (the subject of this chapter), and how skilled we are in applying these resources (detailed in the chapters that follow this one).

We can learn a great deal about current best information sources from librarians and other experts in medical informatics, and should seek hands-on training from them as an essential part of our *clinical* training.

In this chapter we consider the choices and uses of resources that are most likely to provide the best evidence for a given question about the treatment, diagnosis, prognosis, cause, or prevention of a clinical problem. "Best-evidence" resources are built according to an explicit process that values research according to its scientific merit and clinical relevance. You will learn these principles as you go through this book. To be useful for providing the evidence we need for a particular clinical problem, best-evidence resources must be in formats that facilitate rapid searching to find exact matches for clinical questions. Whether the search engine is electronic or a pocket notebook, the important features are portability and easy navigation from clinical questions to evidence-based answers. Fortunately for the readers of this book, this combination of evidence-based content and easy access is now available for a rapidly growing number of health care problems, with vigorous efforts underway to tackle clinical disciplines that are not presently well served. The next part of this chapter provides an orientation to the types of evidence-based sources that exist today. This is followed by opportunities to track down the answers to specific clinical problems.

ORIENTATION TO EVIDENCE-BASED INFORMATION RESOURCES

Where to find the best evidence

1. Burn your (traditional) textbooks

We begin with textbooks only to dismiss them. If the pages of textbooks smelled like decomposing garbage when they get out of date, the unsmelly bits could be useful, because textbooks are generally well organized for clinical use and much of their content will be current at any one time. Unfortunately, there's no way to tell what is up to date and what is not in most texts. So, while we may find some useful information in texts about the pathophysiology of clinical problems, it is best not to use them for establishing the cause, diagnosis, prognosis, prevention or treatment of a disorder.

Having made this bold claim, if we were to burn the textbooks, we would begin to see a phoenix of sorts arising from the ashes. For a textbook to be dependable in the modern era:

- it should be revised frequently (at least once a year)

- it should be heavily referenced, at least for declarations about diagnosis and management (so readers can get to original sources for details and can also easily determine the date of a given claim)

- the evidence in support of a statement should be selected according to explicit principles of evidence.

Only one textbook begins to meet all these criteria at present, *Clinical Evidence*,* first published in 1999 by the BMJ Publishing Group (www.bmjpg.com/index.html) and the American College of Physicians (www.acponline.com). At present, it includes only evidence for treatment of a limited but expanding range of clinical disorders. Other similar texts are on the way, including an exciting book, CD and website called *Evidence-Based on Call* being developed by a worldwide consortium led by a group of recent Oxford graduates <http://cebm.jr2.ox.ac.uk/eboc/eboc.html>.

There are other evidence-based textbook contenders. In the field of general medicine, *UpToDate*, only on CD at present, is updated quarterly, extensively referenced, and provides MEDLINE abstracts for key evidence. This provides the user at least a sporting chance at dating and appraising the supporting evidence. *Scientific American Medicine* also extensively references its contents and this is now augmented by an internet version with links to MEDLINE citations and abstracts, as well as many other web resources. *Harrison's* textbook is also upgrading its currency and provides more references and abstracts on its web version, although the extent of referencing is still very limited. This trend to citation-enriched, web-linked textbooks is encouraging, but none of these texts provides much in the way of systematically

---

* Details of this and most other evidence-based resources mentioned in the chapter are provided in the CD that accompanies the book.

critically appraised evidence, leaving readers to do this for themselves, or to hope that the author has done so. We're also seeing the emergence of more evidence-based specialty texts, such as *Evidence-based Cardiology* from the BMJ Publishing Group. We look forward to many more such texts soon, but beware that these texts are in transition; we need to check to see if the systematic consideration of evidence promised in the title and introduction of these books is actually delivered in the contents.

2. Invest in evidence databases

Although not integrated around clinical problem areas in the convenient way of textbooks, current best evidence from specific studies of clinical problems can be found in an increasing number of electronic databases, some with explicit evidence processing, and some which leave the processing to the user. The best of these at present is Evidence-based Medicine Reviews (EBMR) from Ovid Technologies (www.ovid.com). EBMR combines several electronic databases, including the Cochrane Database of Systematic Reviews, Best Evidence, Evidence-Based Mental Health and Evidence-Based Nursing, Cancerlit, Healthstar, Aidsline, Bioethicsline and MEDLINE, plus links to over 200 full text journals. We've listed the more specialized databases first because, if they are dedicated to the topic area of our interest, we are more likely to find what we want there than in the general database, MEDLINE. EBMR links these databases to one another. Thus, if we find a randomized trial in MEDLINE on a topic of interest, and this trial has been included in a systematic review in the Cochrane Library, the review is just a single keystroke away! EBMR is particularly valuable because of these links from a general database (MEDLINE) to evidence-based services which are prepared according to explicit principles and procedures for sorting evidence according to quality and content. Many health sciences libraries have picked up this service – be sure to check with your library and ask them to get the service if they don't already have it.

The Cochrane Library (CL) (update.cochrane.co.uk; www.update-software.com) and Best Evidence (BE) (www.acponline.org) are also available as separate databases on CD and the internet. CL provides systematic reviews of trials of health care interventions and BE summarizes individual studies and systematic reviews from over 100 medical journals, the studies being selected according to explicit criteria for scientific merit and clinical relevance.

MEDLINE is the world's largest general biomedical research literature database, from basic research through applied. Because MEDLINE was the first medical literature database available to clinicians for electronic searching, many clinicians are now familiar with its use. Because of its huge size (about 10 million references and counting) and broad scope, it has "something for everyone", but it is challenging to get exactly what we want from it. Today, there are more specialized clinical research databases that clinicians may be less familiar with, but which are much easier to use and more likely to yield clinically useful information. The Cochrane Library and Best Evidence are two such databases. As well, MEDLINE "subsets" for clinical practice are prepared by some companies, particularly for the larger specialties such as cardiology. We can also create our own clinical subset by developing a "hedge", or search strategy that narrows searches in MEDLINE to journals that are most likely to provide articles of direct relevance to our own practice. We'll discuss how to do this a bit later. The main message here, however, is that we should look to specialized databases that are tailored for our clinical practice area; MEDLINE should be used as a backup if no such databases exist or if we come up empty-handed on a search of a specialized database. MEDLINE is available for free from many sources, notably its makers, the US National Library of Medicine (www.ncbi.nlm.nih.gov/PubMed). BioMedNet also provides free access to MEDLINE (http://www.biomednet.com) with many enhancements, including links to original sources and related references for each entry.

How to control the evidence that finds you

1. Trade in your (traditional) journal subscriptions

A necessary complement to "look up" databases and texts are "current awareness" services that prompt us when there are important new studies on topics of interest to us. This is the traditional function filled by subscribing to the journals in our field. In the same way that we should burn our (traditional) textbooks, we should trade in our (traditional) journal subscriptions because there are now better resources for keeping current, which are described below.

2. Invest in evidence-based journals and online services

Beginning with *ACP Journal Club* in 1991, a growing number of periodicals summarize the best evidence in traditional journals, making their selections according to explicit criteria for merit, providing structured abstracts of the best studies, and expert commentaries to provide the context of the studies and the clinical applicability of their findings. These new journals include *Evidence-Based Medicine, Evidence-Based Mental Health, Evidence-Based Nursing, Evidence-Based Health Care Policy and Practice*, and *Evidence-Based Cardiovascular Medicine*. These journals do what traditional journals wish they could do in selecting the best studies – traditional journals can't do this because they can only publish from among the articles that authors choose to send them. Thus, these summary journals allow us to do what we couldn't afford to do for ourselves, i.e. summarize the best evidence from high-quality studies selected from all the journals of relevance to our clinical interests.

For the most part, these evidence-based summary journals are targeted for generalists. If you are a subspecialist, you may have to build your own current awareness service. This is easily possible now through having the title pages of journals of relevance to your practice sent to you from such services as Current Contents, MEDLINE, and Silverplatter. Further, subspecialty journal clubs are sprouting on the web, e.g. Peds Journal Club (pedsccm.wustl.edu/EBJournal_club.html), Family Practice JC (POEMS) (www.infopoems.com/POEMS/POEMS_Home.htm), Neurosurgery (http://www.brown.edu/Departments/Neurosurgery/EJC/journ.html), and Critical Care (http://ahsn.lhsc.on.ca). It is difficult to keep track of all the new services. The ones we know about are listed in the CD and will be kept up to date on this book's website (http://www.library.utoronto.ca/medicine/ebm/). SHARR provides excellent links to evidence-based services (www.shef.ac.uk/uni/academic/R-Z/scharr/ir/netting.html).

3. Look into computerized clinical decision support systems

If based on current best evidence, computer information systems that remind us to provide care for specific patients according to their characteristics can improve the care we give.[2] Such information systems are not widely available at present, and the ones that can deliver reminders are often not based on current best evidence, so "buyer beware". But it is technically feasible for machines to match patients' characteristics with evidence-based recommendations that are tailored to them, freeing the patient and care provider to meet the challenge of deciding which recommendations should be implemented and how.

SEARCHING FOR EVIDENCE TO SOLVE PATIENT PROBLEMS

As in swimming and bicycle riding, the use of evidence-based information resources is best illustrated by examples and practice, not by reading. Consider that you are working at the primary care level (don't worry if you're not a primary care clinician – the same basic principles of searching for evidence apply for all clinical disciplines). Commit yourself to paper on three matters for each of the five problems below before you move on to the rest of the chapter:

1. the key question to seek an answer for (using the guidelines from Ch. 1)

2. the best answer to the clinical problem that you currently have stored in your brain (being as quantitative as possible)

3. the evidence resources[†] (both traditional and *avant garde*) that you would consult to find best current answers.

Problem 1

Mr Anders, an accountant, is a moderately obese 56-year-old man with type 2 diabetes, first diagnosed 11 years ago. He is trying to quit his smoking habit of 25 years. No diabetes complications have been

---

† We'll make a distinction here between an evidence resource and an information source. The former reports, or at least cites, original studies or systematic reviews in support of declarations (such as "marmite saves lives"), so that readers can verify the recency, accuracy and applicability of the claim for themselves. The latter may or may not provide evidence in support of claims.

detected so far. His blood sugars are well controlled on metformin but his blood pressure has been mildly elevated, averaging 158/94 mmHg during his past three visits. You propose to prescribe a medication to lower his BP. He has been unable to lower his weight during the past 2 years despite your urgings. He is also not keen to consume additional prescription medication, preferring "natural remedies". He is open to persuasion on the latter, but would like to see the evidence that lowering blood pressure with drugs does more good than harm for people with diabetes and hypertension (the latter of which he figures is just part of the "turf" of his stressful job). As an accountant, he wants to know just how much benefit he can expect for the additional medication we are proposing to prescribe for him.

Write down the key question that identifies the evidence needed to give Mr Anders a clear answer, indicate your best answer before searching (stick your neck out!), and select an evidence resource that you feel will provide current best evidence to support an answer suited to this patient.

Question:

Your best answer (without searching):

Initial evidence resource:

Problem 2

You also find out from Mrs Anders, who accompanies Mr Anders on this visit, that he is taking vitamin E and beta-carotene to lower his risk for heart disease, based on a health advisory that Mrs Anders read on the internet. While looking into the evidence for blood pressure control, you decide to see what you can find on whether these over-the-counter self-treatments reduce the risk for coronary heart disease.

Write down the key question, your "top of the head" answer, and a likely evidence resource:

Question:

Your answer :

Initial evidence resource:

Problem 3

Ms Johnstone-Smythe is a 71-year-old widow with no important health problems until she awakes one morning with right arm clumsiness. She lives with her daughter, who also notes that Mum had garbled speech. On examination, the blood pressure is 154/84 mmHg with a regular heart rate of 72 per minute, you astutely detect a left carotid bruit, and examination of the cardiovascular and neurological systems is otherwise entirely normal. Your diagnosis is a transient ischemic attack (TIA) and you prescribe aspirin. You've recently read about the benefits of carotid endarterectomy, especially for symptomatic high-grade carotid stenosis. On Ms Johnston-Smythe's behalf, you are not keen on referring her for a risky angiogram and would normally order a quick and safe carotid ultrasound, but a colleague of yours recently told you of a similar patient who had a positive carotid ultrasound but a negative angiogram. You don't know whether the ultrasound has a false-negative rate too. You're not really sure how to proceed – ultrasound, then refer if positive, or refer to a specialist right away, and hope for the best. You tell Ms J-S that she may have a narrowing in the artery that leads to the part of her brain that caused the problem earlier in the day, and you refer her to a neurologist straight away – and promise yourself to learn more about how good ultrasound is in detecting (and especially ruling out) treatable carotid lesions, for future reference.

Write down the key question that you need evidence for, the best answer you have currently stored in your brain, and a likely evidence resource:

Question:

Your best answer :

Initial evidence resource:

Problem 4

Mrs Naggan, a 46-year-old woman, has had ulcerative colitis for 7 years now, with extensive involvement of her colon and severe symptoms at times. Her colitis is in remission at present. She is loath to have surgery but is concerned about the mounting risk for cancer that she has heard of through the newsletter of a patient support for her condition. Her spouse has convinced her to find out just what the risk might be.

Write down the key question that you need evidence for, your best answer, and a likely evidence resource:

Question:

Your best answer :

Initial evidence resource:

Problem 5

As part of the compulsory maintenance of competence time that you must account for each year, you audit 150 consecutive patient notes in your practice to determine the proportion of patients for whom you have provided appropriate preventive care. To your dismay, you have been recommending preventive interventions for some patients who are unlikely to be helped and have been missing many patients for whom these interventions are likely to be beneficial. You thought that you had been doing better! You vow to make amends and acquire a copy of the Canadian Task Force on the Periodic Health Examination book.[3] It's 6 years old and 3 inches thick! You can't imagine remembering all of it and wonder if computerized reminders can help you carry out preventive care and other routine tasks.

Write down the key question that you need evidence for, your own answer, and a likely evidence resource:

Question:

Your best answer :

Initial evidence resource:

At this point, you should have written down the key questions, your current answers, and the evidence resources that you feel are best suited to answer these questions. Now would be a good time to try your hand at finding the answers by the routes you've selected, keeping track of how much time, ease/aggravation and money your searches cost and how satisfied you are in the end. Put yourself under some time pressure: summarize the best evidence you can find in 30 minutes or less for each question. (You may be thinking about skipping this exercise, hoping that the rest of this chapter will teach you how to do it effortlessly. But there is wisdom in the maxim "no pain, no gain". Invest at least 30 minutes of your time on at least one of the questions before you press on.)

What follows is a general approach to identifying and using key evidence-based resources, followed by descriptions of various approaches to finding current best evidence to resolve the clinical problems raised above. It is important to note that there may be more than one good route (not to mention a myriad of bad routes), and that as this book ages better routes will assuredly be built. Indeed, many improved resources have become available since publication of the first edition of this book in 1997, including Evidence-Based Medicine Reviews and Clinical Evidence, while others, such as the Cochrane Library, have greatly matured. Thus, one of the foundations of providing evidence-based health care is keeping tabs on the availability, scope and quality of any new resources that are directly pertinent to our own professional practice. If you have tried to search for evidence on these problems, compare what you did and what you found with our methods. If you haven't tried to search yet, we issue you a challenge: see if you can find a better answer than we did (we searched in early 1999, but we won't begrudge you a better answer that you found after this time). Updates on effective searching strategies, including especially those that our readers create, will appear (with attribution) on this book's website (http://www.library.utoronto.ca/medicine/ebm/).

CARRYING OUT THE SEARCHING STEPS

Basic steps for acquiring the evidence to support a clinical decision appear in Figure 2.1. We've supplied the clinical problems, and have asked you to take the first step, defining the questions to be answered, following the lead in Chapter 1. Have a go at it if you haven't done so already. Here's our try for the first example above.

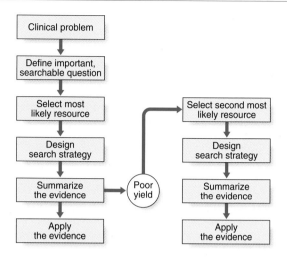

Figure 2.1 General search strategy.

Problem 1 Efficacy of aggressive blood pressure lowering in diabetes mellitus

The clinical problem The diabetic man with hypertension.

Step 1. Asking an answerable question

> In a 56-year-old man with type 2 diabetes mellitus and untreated hypertension, does "tight" blood pressure control reduce subsequent morbidity and mortality?

Step 2A. Selecting an evidence resource

Step 2A is to decide where to search. The examples in this chapter are drawn from the authors' clinical practice of internal medicine, so the focus will be on the best and quickest evidence-based information sources for internal medicine, including general and specialized bibliographic databases, in both print and electronic form. For completeness, we'll also take a look at traditional textbooks (that we suggested you burn earlier in the chapter) and texts that are making the transition to citing supportive evidence, to see how they fare. For the most part, electronic media with periodic updates, whether on the internet, computer disk, or CD-ROM, are rendering paper sources obsolete for looking up evidence, although paper journals still play an important role in alerting practitioners to new evidence as it becomes available ("current awareness"). Electronic media are generally much more accessible, much more thoroughly indexed, and, most importantly, have the potential to be much more up to date. Moreover, hypertext and the internet permit unlimited linkages to related and supplementary information. Thus, a good computer (whether ours or someone else's!),‡ with a fast modem or internet link and a compact disk (CD) drive, and a working knowledge of the evidence resources that have been developed for our own clinical discipline, can make an important difference to whether we will be successful in becoming evidence-based practitioners.§

For blood pressure control in type 2 diabetes mellitus, we will begin with a new resource, Evidence-Based Medicine Reviews (EBMR). Described earlier in this chapter, this service links several evidence-based databases, and is currently the most comprehensive evidence-based service available. As a result, it will most often be the premier resource for one-stop shopping. That will not necessarily make it the best resource for a given question, but it is the right place to start if you don't know exactly what is the best source, and you have access to it. As mentioned earlier, EBMR is available in many health sciences libraries (often at no charge to the user) and on the internet (for a price).

Step 2B. Executing the search strategy

Once the choice of resource has been made, the next step is to design a search strategy. Starting with the Best Evidence

---

‡ One of us was on a medical school committee a decade ago considering whether we should require all students to have their own computer. We said no because, after looking at the software of the day, we concluded that there were no useful clinical applications worth having. How times change!

§ If you are computerless, make friends with a librarian; if you are computer-phobic, sign up for desensitization right away!

(BE) database in EBMR, a search on "diabetes mellitus and hypertension" yields 112 references – far too many to scroll through. If we add "and randomized controlled trial" to this search we end up with a manageable 19 references. The search takes about 3 minutes, including sign-in to the Ovid service on the internet.

Step 2C. Examining the evidence summary

Judging by its short title, the third reference retrieved from the EBMR search of BE appears to be right on target – "Review: Several interventions reduce complications in type 2 diabetes mellitus", a specially prepared abstract and commentary on the systematic reviews of evidence on diabetes care by Vijan et al.[4] The Best Evidence abstract tells us:

Antihypertensive therapy reduces mortality in persons with diabetes, and a target blood pressure of 130/85 has been recommended by experts. Only low-dose diuretics have been directly shown to decrease mortality in persons with diabetes. Angiotensin-converting enzyme (ACE) inhibitors (in patients with nephropathy) and beta-blockers (after myocardial infarction) may have other specific benefits.

With a relatively small and select database like BE (just over 1200 references compared with over millions in MEDLINE and EMBASE), it is very easy to find things.

If you happen to have BE on your personal computer, the search, using the terms "hypertension and diabetes", restricted to studies on therapy, takes about 22 seconds, yielding the same key reference (no surprise) plus a bonus: a study that shows that diuretics reduced major cardiovascular events in elderly hypertensive diabetics compared with placebo (20 vs. 28%, respectively, number needed to treat, 13**).[5]

We might have stopped at this point, but the abstract for the article by Vijan et al[4] didn't provide quantitative information about the benefits of lowering blood pressure in type 2 diabetes and the commentary by Leiter alluded to trials in

---

** The number needed to treat is defined on page 113.

progress at the time, in 1997. Switching to the MEDLINE database in EBMR, selecting the period 1996 to the present, to see if there are more recent references, we enter the following individual search terms: (1) "hypertension" (10 274 "hits"); (2) "diabetes mellitus, non-insulin dependent" (4808 hits); and (3) "clinical trial (publication type)" (53 918 hits). Combining these terms ("1 and 2 and 3") yields 63 references. The much greater size of the database is immediately apparent in the number of hits. Predictably, most of the additional references will be of no interest for this query; however, the proportion of "false drops" (a term that librarians use that is equivalent to "false positives") in MEDLINE searches is typically about 90%, so most of what you retrieve from this source is "junk", at least for the question you are attempting to answer.

Nevertheless, in this particular search, the first 10 references retrieved yield some gold. The best nuggets are three reports from the United Kingdom Prospective Diabetes Study,[6-8] which showed that intensive BP control among moderately hypertensive patients with type 2 diabetes led to a relative risk reduction of

24% in diabetes related end points (95% confidence interval 8% to 38%) (P=0.0046), 32% in deaths related to diabetes (6% to 51%) (P = 0.019), 44% in strokes (11% to 65%) (P = 0.013), and 37% in microvascular end points (11% to 56%) (P = 0.0092), predominantly owing to a reduced risk of retinal photocoagulation.

Enalapril had similar benefits to atenolol but patients were more likely to continue to take enalapril.[7] Furthermore, aggressive treatment was cost-effective.[8]

Many health sciences libraries provide access to the EBMR service at no cost to the user. Individual subscriptions to EBMR are relatively expensive, however, at US$795 at the time of writing. This is for a single user license, which could easily serve a large clinic.

Application of the evidence

After satisfying yourself that the evidence is valid, important, and applicable to your patient, you discuss hypertension management with Mr Anders, indicating that these are important new findings. He agrees to a trial of enalapril.

Comments

The Cochrane Library provides access to systematic reviews and yields 741 articles indexed with the term "diabetes and hypertension". Browsing through the hits in the Cochrane Database of Systematic Reviews (one of four databases in the Cochrane Library) you soon come to a Cochrane review entitled "Antihypertensive therapy in diabetes mellitus".[9] This review concludes that treating hypertension produces benefits for both primary and secondary prevention, but that this is based on diabetes subgroup analyses from trials of treating hypertension, not trials specifically designed for patients with diabetes and hypertension. The first page of the review indicates that it was last updated in August 1997. This review was clearly out of date when we searched in the Cochrane Library, Issue 1 for 1999, missing the new landmark UKPDS studies of antihypertensive care among patients with type 2 diabetes. These studies were also not included in the remaining 740 references on hypertension and diabetes, although many other 1998 citations were included. It is obvious that a time-lag exists between publication of an original study in a journal and when it can be included in any database service, including MEDLINE (which will lag by 3–6 months for priority journals), Best Evidence (which will lag by 6 months), and the Cochrane Library (which will have a variable lag, depending on the schedule for updating the Cochrane Clinical Trials Registry and individual reviews). Resource users need to take this into account, especially when patients come expecting your views on the latest word they have heard from press versions of studies that are released on the day before their first publication in traditional journals! The fastest route in this particular situation is to go right to the website for the journal. The UKPDS studies are all available in full text at the BMJ website (www.bmjpg.com), being posted to the web on the day preceding print publication.

The time-lag from first publication to incorporation into secondary resources means that, for new treatments, it is usually a waste of time to consult a print textbook, unless it has been very recently released. Even for printed books, months pass between when chapters are written and when the print version is released. CD-ROM texts can improve on this if frequently updated. *UpToDate in Medicine*, volume 6, issue 3 for 1998 was right up to date for hypertension management in diabetes, providing details of the UKPDS trials.[10] *Harrison's Principles of Internal of Medicine* CD-ROM[11] had very little on the treatment of hypertension among diabetics and didn't include recent references on this topic. The January 1999 CD-ROM issue of *Scientific American Medicine* (*SAM*)[12] had several hits for hypertension and diabetes but didn't provide specific information or references concerning tight BP control. *SAM* did, however, provide web links for subscribers; in this case, the link led to a key resource with evidence-based – but somewhat dated – guidelines on the treatment of hypertension in patients with diabetes mellitus.[13] The January 1999 issue of the *SAM* CD was out of date for diabetes and hypertension, but provided more information than *Harrison's*, and has the chance, which *Harrison's* lacks, to make amends with its monthly print and quarterly disk updates. The *Oxford Textbook of Medicine*[14] was out of date for hypertension in diabetes. Kumar and Clark's *Clinical Medicine*, 3rd edition[15] had a short section advising aggressive treatment of hypertension for patients with diabetic nephropathy (found through the index under hypertension, not under diabetes).

Even print resources can be up to date if they are issued frequently and maintained properly. *Clinical Evidence* has an excellent, evidence-based chapter on managing diabetes, including the key studies on blood pressure control. Thus, the take home message is that we need to know how a text, CD, or internet site is constructed to ensure that important new advances are incorporated quickly. Failing that, the resource should at least provide references for key content so we can discern the date of publication of the evidence that is cited.

Problem 2 Efficacy of vitamin E and beta-carotene: friends, foes, or just more fees?

The clinical problem The smoker at high risk for cardiovascular disease.

Step 1. Asking an answerable question

> In high cardiovascular risk male smokers, do vitamin E and carotene prevent clinical events or death?

Step 2A. Selecting an evidence resource + Step 2B. Executing the search strategy

A quick search (30 seconds) of Best Evidence 3 for "vitamin E and beta-carotene" retrieved 11 items, including several large randomized trials.

Step 2C. Examining the evidence summary

Best Evidence contains only studies that have been pre-appraised for scientific validity and pre-screened for clinical relevance. Thus, once you've determined that the study you've retrieved is on target for the patient's question you need to solve, you can elect to skip the report's methodology, especially if you discern, right at the start (from the title, for example), that the treatment doesn't work. Scanning the findings of the vitamin E and beta-carotene trials, you quickly discover that vitamin E had, at best, a small effect in reducing the incidence of angina[16] but that beta-carotene actually increases the risk of myocardial infarction recurrence among smokers. Further, neither drug reduced the risk for cancer, and beta-carotene increased the risk for lung cancer among smokers.[17, 18]

Application of the evidence

After satisfying yourself that the evidence is valid, important, and applicable to your patient, you discuss it with Mr and Mrs Anders and suggest that the new antihypertensive drug that will benefit Mr Anders be substituted for the beta-carotene, which may harm him. You advise him to give up smoking in any event and offer him strategies to help (the evidence for which is readily retrieved from a 30-second search of BE on "smoking cessation"). For Mrs Anders, you offer her internet addresses where she can do more research on home remedies and medical treatments (www.nlm.nih.gov/medlineplus – set up by the US National Library of Medicine specially for the public), and guidelines (www.guideline.gov). On the way home, you drop by your local pharmacy and are amazed to observe that beta-carotene is on prominent display, to be sold over-the-counter, and with no warnings whatsoever about adverse effects on its label. You wonder about the justice of people spending more money on non-prescription drugs like this than on prescriptions and try your luck at convincing the pharmacist to rethink this display.

Comments

UpToDate has an excellent section on the antioxidants vitamin E and beta-carotene, including the evidence that beta-carotene may be harmful for smokers. A MEDLINE search through the Clinical Queries service of PubMed (http://www.ncbi.nlm.nih.gov/clinicnal.html), searching on "vitamin E and beta-carotene" and using a specific search filter for randomized controlled trials produced 279 references. No major trials appeared in the first page of 20 references – almost time to move on, but persistence pays: the Rapola study was 21st on the list. *Harrison's* and *SAM* also cited two trials with adverse effects from beta-carotene in lung cancer prevention, but neither provided findings for cardiovascular disease. A Cochrane Library search on beta-carotene retrieved no reviews in the Cochrane Database of Systematic Reviews, one outdated non-Cochrane review in its Database of Abstracts of Reviews of Evidence, and many trial and review references in the Cochrane Clinical Trials Register.

The search filters that are used in PubMed Clinical Queries are designed to improve the yield of searches for clinically relevant and scientifically sound studies, increasing the yield of useful studies and reducing the yield of false drops.[19] These strategies are reproduced in Table 2.1. In each case, the best single term to filter the search for studies of treatment, prognosis, etiology and diagnosis is provided, followed by a more complex search strategy that provides a better filter. It is a good idea to keep the single terms handy when searching MEDLINE through access routes other than PubMed Clinical Queries; in PubMed you can put the more complex strategies to work simply by clicking on both the "category" (therapy etc.) and "emphasis" (sensitivity or specificity) buttons. If you want a few good references without a lot of false drops, click on

Table 2.1 Best single terms and combinations for high-sensitivity MEDLINE searches for the best studies of treatment, diagnosis, prognosis, or cause

Search strategy	Sensitivity[a]	Specificity[a]	Precision[a]
For studies of prevention or treatment			
Clinical trial (pt)	0.93	0.92	0.49
Randomized controlled trial (pt) or Drug therapy (sh) or Therapeutic use (sh) or Random: (tw)	0.99	0.74	0.22
For studies of prognosis			
Exp cohort studies	0.60	0.80	0.11
Incidence or Exp mortality or Follow-up studies or Mortality (sh) or Prognosis: (tw) or Predict: (tw) or Course (tw)	0.92	0.73	0.11
For studies of etiology or cause			
Risk (tw)	0.67	0.79	0.15
Exp cohort studies or Exp risk or Odds and ratio: (tw) or Relative and risk (tw) or Case and control: (tw)	0.82	0.70	0.14
For studies of diagnosis			
Diagnosis& (pe)	0.80	0.77	0.09
Exp sensitivity a#d specificity or Diagnosis& (pe) or Diagnostic use or Sensitivity (tw) or Specificity (tw)	0.92	0.73	0.09

[a] Sensitivity here is the proportion of studies in MEDLINE meeting criteria for scientific soundness and clinical relevance that are detected. Specificity is the proportion of less sound/relevant studies that are excluded by the search strategy. Precision is the proportion of all citations retrieved that are both sound and relevant.

"specificity". If you want an exhaustive search, or don't find anything you want in the specific search, click on "sensitivity".

Another valuable feature of PubMed is the "[See Related Articles]" tag that appears after each citation you retrieve. If your search finds an article that meets your needs and you would like to see some more on the same topic, clicking on this link retrieves additional related articles.

Problem 3 Diagnosis of carotid stenosis

The clinical problem Determining operability following a transient ischemic attack.

Step 1. Asking an answerable question

In a 71-year-old woman with a recent left hemispheric transient ischemic attack, is carotid ultrasound a trustworthy intermediate step to angiography in diagnosing surgically remediable carotid stenosis?

Step 2A. Selecting an evidence resource

UpToDate has done well in the first two problems, so let's look at it again for this problem. If no luck there, we'll try Best Evidence, and move to MEDLINE if BE doesn't pay off.

Step 2B. Executing the search strategy

A search on "carotid stenosis" in *UpToDate* leads in about 50 seconds to a section on "evaluation of carotid artery stenosis". A lot of information is presented here, with a stated preparation date just 6 months before we did the search. The authors provide some pros and cons of various methods and quote some individual studies of non-invasive tests, but no methods for selecting these studies are reported and no comment on the quality of the methods of the studies is provided. It is not clear in reading the text what the best approach would be. This may be the state of the art, but how can one tell? Let's seek some verification from another source.

A search on Best Evidence 3 on "carotid", restricted to studies of diagnosis, took about 15 seconds and provided several references including a meta-analysis of studies of non-invasive tests for carotid stenosis compared with angiography published in MEDLINE between 1977 and 1993.[20] For carotid duplex ultrasonography, the sensitivities and specificities for detecting 70% internal carotid stenosis were 88% and about 90%, respectively. While these figures are quite high, they mean that some patients would still be falsely labeled as above or below 70% stenosis. But since the most recent studies reviewed were published in 1993, these figures might be out of date and ultrasonography may have improved since then.

Extending the search to PubMed Clinical Queries, searching on "carotid endarterectomy", and using the filter for "diagnosis", emphasizing "specificity", 165 citations were retrieved. It took over half an hour to construct and run this search and appraise the findings by scanning titles, and assessing the abstracts for articles with promising titles. An article by Criswell et al[21] reported a comparison of the same model of duplex scanner in two different hospitals; the results were significantly different, documenting a problem in the reproducibility of the test results. A second study, by Bain et al,[22] investigated only those patients in whom high-grade stenosis was found on duplex ultrasonography. Thus, it provided no information on patients who might have had false-negative findings on ultrasonography. Nevertheless, the study did provide interesting information about how well the ultrasonography obviated the need for angiography:

Duplex imaging was not able to predict accurately which arteriograms would provide useful additional information [sensitivity 59%, specificity 65%] [compared with arteriograms], whereas 89 arteriograms [33%] contained information [not found on US] that might have influenced subsequent management.

(We have added information in square parentheses for clarity.)

During your searching on MEDLINE, you decide to see if there is anything on the value of the clinical observation that you made, that your patient had a carotid bruit. You search on "carotid stenosis and auscultation", which retrieves 54 documents. One of these reports that a focal ipsilateral carotid bruit had a sensitivity of 63% and a specificity of 61% for high-grade stenosis and, when absent, only lowered the probability for high-grade stenosis from a pre-test value of 52% to a post-test probability of 40%.[23]

Step 2C. Examining the evidence summary

You conclude that neither listening for an ipsilateral bruit nor carrying out a duplex ultrasound can rule in or rule out high-grade carotid stenosis. You feel a bit deflated to learn that the bruit you had boasted to one of your colleagues about finding is so insensitive and non-specific. (There is more about sensitivity and specificity in Ch. 3.)

Application of the evidence

While it would be nice to be able to assure patients with TIAs or minor strokes that a simple non-invasive test could indicate whether they might benefit from surgery, you decide to tell such patients for whom surgery might be indicated that you cannot spare them a referral for further testing and that they will likely need to have an angiogram.

Problem 4 Prognosis of ulcerative colitis

The clinical problem Determining the risk of subsequent cancer in a patient with ulcerative colitis.

Step 1. Asking an answerable question

In a 46-year-old woman with a 7-year history of extensive ulcerative colitis, what is the risk for developing bowel cancer?

Step 2A. Selecting an evidence resource

Ulcerative colitis is a fairly common chronic disease and its prognosis ought to be accurately and consistently represented in textbooks of medicine. Let's give the texts another chance!

Step 2B. Executing the search strategy

A survey of some of the most popular textbooks of medicine belies the charitable notion that they should provide consistent and quantitative information on prognosis and complications. Kumar and Clark's *Clinical Medicine*[15] states that "In ulcerative colitis the risk of carcinoma of the colon in a patient who has had total colitis for more than 10 years is much greater than it is for the general population" (p. 220). Jewell, in the *Oxford Textbook of Medicine*,[14] does not cite a reference but indicates that, "The most recent series studying primary cohorts suggest that the cumulative risk for patients with extensive disease is about 7 to 15 per cent at 20 years, with very little risk up to 15 years of disease" (p. 1950). The *Harrison's* CD, however, provides more details. A search on "ulcerative colitis and cancer" within 10 words of each other retrieves eight chapter references, the most useful of which appears to be a chapter on inflammatory bowel disease, which appears in seventh spot on the retrieval list. Clicking on this "hit" leads to three references from the medical literature at the end of the chapter. The first reference is just a citation, but the second includes an abstract of a community-based study.[24] This report of a cohort of patients with ulcerative colitis in Sweden indicated that the relative risk for cancer was increased 14.8-fold (95% confidence interval, 11.4–18.9) for patients with extensive colitis at onset overall, but that this risk was reduced to about 3.7 times if onset was in the 30–39 year age period (as for our patient). The duration of follow-up wasn't stated in the abstract and we would need to check the complete article to determine this, as well as whether the cohort was of patients at first diagnosis ("inception cohort"), and whether the follow-up was adequate. The text of Glickman's chapter in *Harrison's* provides additional detail, stating that:

It has been estimated that with pancolitis there is a risk of cancer of 12% at 15 years, 23% at 20 years, and 42% at 24 years, although estimates in community practices have been lower, with the probability that colon cancer will develop in patients with pancolitis being 10% at 26 years.

Forty-two per cent at 24 years vs. 10% at 26 years … . Hmmm … seems like a rather remarkable difference in risk estimates, but no studies are cited in support of either figure (the references above being in a bibliography at the end of the chapter, not cited in the text) so we'll have to look elsewhere to sort out why these differences have arisen. As set out at the beginning of this chapter, we're seeing this patient at the "community practice" level – but she has certainly seen a specialist when her colitis has flared. What do we tell her? We'll need to press on if we want to get to the bottom of this.

The same search was run on the *SAM* CD, yielding a section of similar length to that in *Harrison's*, including the following statement: "The cumulative risk that cancer of the colon will develop becomes substantial after eight to 10 years of ulcerative colitis, ranging from three percent after 15 years to nine percent after 25 years".[25] The text goes on to give pancolitis as a factor increasing the risk. The figures cited by *SAM* are backed by a reference. This suggests that the figures might be based on evidence that has been carefully collected, but it cannot be assumed that this is so. More detail on the cited study can be garnered from PubMed. The citation and its abstract are easily retrieved by the handy "citation matcher" that appears as a menu item on the opening screen, searching for "Lennard-Jones JE" and "1990", the year of the citation in *SAM*. The abstract is on target but not fully convincing. A total of 401 patients with extensive ulcerative colitis were studied during a 22-year period, with only nine lost to follow-up because they moved from the country. Patients had sigmoidoscopy and biopsy at follow-up visits; when the patient's course had reached 10 years, colonoscopy was done every 2 years. It is very likely that this is a "referral" population, not community-based, but it is unclear from the abstract whether it is an "inception cohort" of patients who were all followed from very early on in their illness, a key requirement for the valid assessment of prognosis (see Ch. 3). There is also no information in the abstract about cancer rates in the general community that would be needed to determine the magnitude of any increase in risk. We will either have to retrieve and appraise the whole article or try another route to evidence.

We conducted an additional search in the "advanced search" section of PubMed, on "ulcerative colitis AND neoplasm AND cohort studies". This retrieved 243 articles, a daunting number, but several near the beginning of the retrieval proved to be well done studies. Palli et al[26] reported that mortality, if anything, was less than expected compared with population rates, even though cancer of the bowel was somewhat increased. Using the "[See Related Articles]" link led to the article by Ekbom et al[24] cited in *Harrison's*. Stewenius et al[27] reported a population-based study in which there was a 30% increase in mortality compared with the general population, and an incidence of colorectal cancer of 2.1 times that in age- and sex-specific rates in the city, but the absolute risk for colorectal cancer was very low at 1.4 cases per 1000 patient-years. A Danish population-based study gave a similar figure for relative risk of 1.8.[28]

Best Evidence provides a fast check and has one study directly on target. A Danish study[29] followed an inception cohort of adults with ulcerative colitis, based on all cases in a county (i.e. the study was population-based), and with 99.9% follow-up. The study reported no increase in the risk for cancer compared with the general Danish population, but this appears to have been in the context of a close surveillance program with a substantial colectomy rate: 24% at 10 years and 32% at 25 years. There was an increase in mortality compared with the general population only during the first year after diagnosis. The commentator for the study indicated that the study was well done, but that the colectomy rate was quite high, especially for patients with pancolitis (39%), and that this may be the reason for the absence of an increased risk for colon cancer.

Step 2C. Examining the evidence summary

Population-based studies documented a small increase in cancer risk in ulcerative colitis, especially in patients with severe or extensive colitis, but the absolute risk was low: <10% at 20 years. With regular follow-up and an aggressive approach to colectomy, it appears that the risk for colon cancer might be reduced, but there is at least one skeptical group.[30] As the indications for colectomy are several (failure of intensive drug therapy, toxic megacolon, debilitating extracolonic manifestations, as well as the suspicion of cancer in a stricture), it would be very difficult to conduct a randomized trial of colectomy vs. observation to distinguish truly low risk from the effects of selective colectomy. This is a common problem in studying prognosis: there are very few disorders for which medical interventions do not "interfere" with studying the natural history of the condition. This is fine if the treatments work – but it is difficult to be sure without properly designed trials.

Application of the evidence

We're not sure what to tell the patient at this point. Certainly it would do to reassure her that the period of increased risk for death (the first year) has passed. It is not clear whether colonoscopy every other year beginning at 10 years would be a good idea. No case has been made for prophylactic colectomy. Any other attention to her bowel should be based on her symptoms.

Comments

The risk for colon cancer stated in *Harrison's* 14th edition was frankly confusing – it wasn't backed up by a reference to evidence and none of the studies we looked at directly supported the high rate reported. *SAM* provided some evidence, but the quality of the evidence wasn't clear. A textbook of gastroenterology would certainly provide more detail than a general medical textbook – but primary care physicians, who provide our perspective for this chapter, would likely not have many current specialty texts close at hand (the internet will provide the solution to this problem in due course).

The MEDLINE literature searches we conducted were messy and time-consuming, but provided some consistent evidence on the increased, but quite low-level, risk for colorectal cancer among patients with long-standing ulcerative colitis. Best Evidence was quick, and provided reassuring evidence that low cancer risk could be achieved, but was inconclusive about how this was done.

Problem 5 Usefulness of computerized reminder systems for preventive care

The clinical problem Computer reminders in preventive medicine.

Step 1. Asking an answerable question

In ambulatory practice, can computerized reminder systems improve the quality of preventive care?

Step 2A. Selecting an evidence resource

Let's look for a systematic review in EBMR reviews.

Step 2B. Executing the search strategy

We started with "reminders" and were deftly guided by the Ovid software into "reminder systems". We selected the options provided of "exploding" this term (to include all of its "subheadings") and making it the "focus" of the article. This gave 62 references, so we clicked on "Limit to EBM Reviews". Two articles survived this weeding out and the second of these was right on target.[31] We clicked on the highlighted "Article Review" at the end of the citation and linked to its abstract and commentary in Evidence-Based Medicine.[32]

For the sake of completeness, we tried a different approach in the MEDLINE database: "preventive medicine and software". This retrieved three citations, two of which are right on target.[2, 33]

Step 2C. Evidence synthesis

The article by Shea et al[31] indicated that computer reminders and manual reminder systems both improve the likelihood that preventive care interventions will be administered in a timely fashion. Although computer reminders appeared to be a little more effective than manual reminders, the difference wasn't statistically significant. Hunt et al's[2] report is more recent, with literature searching to March 1998, and provided similar evidence for computer reminders (manual reminder systems were not considered). The study by Overhage et al[33] tested computer reminders for preventive care among in-patients in an acute hospital: of interest, even though clinicians felt this would be a timely way to provide preventive care, reminders did not increase the rate of implementation.

Application of the evidence

We decided to develop a manual system for reminders for preventive care, according to a chart of preventive care indications from the US. We started to assemble a list of preventive care recommendations by consulting the National Guideline Clearinghouse on the web (www.guideline.gov), but quickly realized that it provides a lot of detailed guidelines on individual conditions, without providing an integrated overview. Further, the Clearinghouse provides recommendations on the same topic from more than one organization, often several. It provides an intriguing mechanism to compare recommendations from two or more guidelines – but the task of going through hundreds of guidelines and comparing across recommendations on the same guideline is more than any of us can bear. We decided to look in a textbook in the hope that someone has done this for us. A search in *SAM* quickly revealed a chapter on preventive health care that compared guidelines by the US and Canadian national task forces on preventive care, as well as the American College of Physicians Clinical Efficacy Assessment Program, organized in a way that made implementation relatively straightforward. Our only reservation was that the chapter was last updated in December 1996. (*Harrison's* had a similar chapter, while the information in *UpToDate* on prevention was much more limited.)

CURRENT AWARENESS: A COMPLEMENT TO PROBLEM-SOLVING

Our focus in this chapter has been on information services that permit us to look up evidence concerning clinical problems that we need to solve in "real time", i.e. it was "necessity-driven". These resources for problem-solving are essential to evidence-based care. But how do we know when our general knowledge base is rendered obsolete by new evidence?[††] Keeping up to date is the traditional role of journal reading and all surveys of physicians indicate that journal reading is the first activity we name in keeping

---

[††] As Will Rogers, an American cowboy philosopher, put it, "It ain't so much what we don't know that gets us into trouble but what we do know that ain't so."

current – but we devote so little time per week to this task that it is impossible to believe that we are doing a good job!

Fortunately, several "summary" or "survey" publications are available, or in the works, that provide abstracts or summaries of key articles of importance to practitioners of various clinical persuasions. Unfortunately, not all of them protect us from studies that are misleading or invalid. There are two basic principles that any summary journal must observe if it is to relieve us of the burden of trying to browse through primary journals ourselves (an activity we not only don't do, but can't do, as we learned back in the Introduction). First, the summary publications should provide explicit criteria for seeking and selecting the studies that will be featured, so that readers will know which journals have been covered and how articles have been selected from these journals. Second, these survey journals (or survey sections in original journals) should report enough information about the methods of the studies they review that readers can judge for themselves their quality and applicability to their own patients, i.e. they should be "evidence-driven". At present, at least five journals meet these criteria, *ACP Journal Club* (for major studies in internal medicine, family medicine, psychiatry, surgery, obstetrics, gynecology, and pediatrics); *Evidence-Based Medicine* (with similar coverage to *ACP Journal Club*); *Evidence-Based Mental Health*; *Evidence-Based Nursing*; *Evidence-Based Cardiovascular Medicine*; and *Journal of Evidence-Based Healthcare*. Sections in the *Journal of Pediatrics* and the *Clinical Journal of Sport Medicine* also provide this type of service. Table 2.2 summarizes the effect of applying the "evidence-driven" and clinical relevance criteria to a selection of journals from the perspective of internal medicine. As shown in this table, even the five best journals yield just one article for every two issues! No wonder it is impossible to keep up with the primary literature: a lot of time is wasted just finding the handful of studies worth paying attention to!

If there are no secondary evidence-based publications in your own field of interest, a fall-back position is to use the criteria from one of the evidence-based journals and determine the yield of clinically important articles in the primary journals in

Table 2.2 Where's the meat in clinical journals? Top 20 journals contributing to *ACP Journal Club* (general internal medicine) in the period 1994–98,[a] ordered by number of articles that met validity criteria

Journal	No. (%) of articles abstracted in *ACP Journal Club* 1994–98	Approximate percentage of journal's articles with abstracts that passed criteria
N Engl J Med	147 (20)	12.6
JAMA	101 (13)	7.2
Lancet	94 (13)	6.2
Ann Intern Med	82 (11)	7.6
BMJ	61 (8)	4.4
Arch Intern Med	46 (6)	2.4
Circulation	27 (4)	1.7
Am J Med	8 (1)	1.1
J Intern Med	5 (1)	1.2
Others[b]	179 (24)	<0.1
Total	750 (100)	

[a] Does not include the Cochrane Database of Systematic Reviews.

[b] Journals with two to four articles abstracted: *Stroke* (4), *J Am J Cardiol* (4), *J Gen Intern Med* (4), *Neurology* (3), *Diabetes Care* (3), *Gastroenterology* (2), *CMAJ* (2), *J Am Geriatric Soc* (2).

your own field. That is, use the same validity criteria plus your own relevance criteria and create your own version of Table 2.2. Then concentrate your journal subscriptions and reading on the journals at the top of the list. For most clinical fields this will be a combination of the four or five largest circulation general journals and a small number of specialty journals. Then, as you scan them, use the validity criteria to select the few articles worth reading – as we'll show you in the next five chapters of this book, you often can accept or reject an article in a few seconds just by looking at its abstract.

It's worth noting that we can learn more by devoting our scarce reading time to working in the "necessity-driven" mode, looking for evidence to solve specific clinical problems, than we will by browsing through low-yield primary journals for evidence that we hope we will be able to recall when we need it later. Balance is called for, and the authors of this book devote 50–75% of their reading time to articles tracked down in solving clinical problems rather than devoutly reading clinical journals.

PARTING SHOTS

MEDLINE is the most sensitive source of current evidence (both "best" and "not so good") at present because of its breadth and constant maintenance. Pre-appraised sources, such as the Cochrane Library and Best Evidence, provide the most specific highway to the best evidence. Evidence-Based Medicine Reviews, by combining the latter with MEDLINE, provides the best opportunity with a single "log-in" to date to find evidence that has been pre-appraised for methods and clinical content when it is available, with instant access to the general medical literature when it is not. It is still important to evidence-based practice that clinicians develop and hone MEDLINE searching skills and acquire local access. All MEDLINE systems are drawn from the same database, prepared by the US National Library of Medicine, but the vendors of MEDLINE offer a variety of subsets, including ones developed for specific clinical practice groups.

MEDLINE has important limitations for clinical use, however, and databases of subsets of articles relevant for clinical practice are needed to make electronic searching for evidence quicker and more fruitful. Fortunately, the technology for close-to-instant access is widely available, and databases with high-quality content are beginning to emerge with disk, CD-ROM and online access. We've looked at some early entrants in this chapter. New services are being developed at a rapid clip so keep your eyes peeled (we will, too, and will cite them on the website for this book: http://www.library.utoronto.ca/medicine/ebm/)! And don't accept anything that doesn't cite the original evidence in support of its assertions (a dictum which, we guess, is the literature equivalent of "Don't take any wooden nickels").

Are textbooks obsolete? Their bloated girth and the rapid obsolescence of their action parts on diagnosis, prognosis and especially therapy make it difficult to believe that they will survive the electronic age any better that dinosaurs did the ice age (although, by analogy, they retain an aesthetic charm for many in their frozen form). Nevertheless, textbooks do integrate information from a wide range of sources, something the time-challenged reader may be unable to do. A new super-breed of text may be on the way, with explicit criteria for selecting evidence, a credible evidence search process, and citation of evidence to support recommendations. *Clinical Evidence* is promising in this respect and *UpToDate*, if it became more explicit about its evidence processing, could fit the bill as well.

References

1 Quote in Pickering G W. BMJ 1956; 2: 113–6.

2 Hunt D L, Haynes R B, Hanna S E, Smith K. Effects of computer-based clinical decision support systems on physician performance and patient outcomes: a systematic review. JAMA 1998; 280: 1339–46.

3 Canadian Task Force on Periodic Health Examination. Canadian guide to clinical preventive health care. Communication Publishing, Ottawa, 1994.

4 Vijan S, Stevens D L, Herman W H, Funnell M M, Standiford C J. Screening, prevention, counseling, and treatment for the complications of type II diabetes mellitus. Putting evidence into practice. J Gen Intern Med 1997; 12: 567–80.

5 Curb J D, Pressel S L, Cutler J A, et al, for the Systolic Hypertension in the Elderly Program Cooperative Research Group. Effect of diuretic-based antihypertensive treatment on cardiovascular disease risk in older diabetic patients with isolated systolic hypertension. JAMA 1996; 276: 1886–92.

6 UK Prospective Diabetes Study Group. Tight blood pressure control and risk of macrovascular and microvascular complications in type 2 diabetes: UKPDS 38. BMJ 1998; 317: 703–13.

7 UK Prospective Diabetes Study Group. Efficacy of atenolol and captopril in reducing risk of macrovascular and microvascular complications in type 2 diabetes: UKPDS 39. BMJ 1998; 317: 713–20.

8 UK Prospective Diabetes Study Group. Cost effectiveness analysis of improved blood pressure control in hypertensive patients with type 2 diabetes: UKPDS 40. BMJ 1998; 317: 720–6.

9 Fuller J, Stevens L K, Chaturvedi N, Holloway J F. Antihypertensive therapy in diabetes mellitus (Cochrane Review). In: The Cochrane Library, Issue 1, 1999. Update Software, Oxford

10 UpToDate in Medicine, Wellesley, MA, USA, BDR Inc. UpToDate, PO Box 812098, Wellesley, MA 02181-0013, USA. Serial CD-ROM. Vol 6, No 3, 1998.

11 Fauci A S, Braunwald E, Isselbacher K J et al (eds) Harrison's principles of internal medicine, 14th edn, version 1.1 (CD ROM). McGraw-Hill, Philadelphia, 1998.

12 SAM-CD. Scientific American Medicine – CD. Dale DC, Federman DG (eds). New York: Scientific American Medicine. Serial CD-ROM. January 1999.

13 Joint National Committee on Prevention, Detection, Evaluation, and Treatment of High Blood Pressure. Sixth report. NIH Publication No. 98-4080. National Institutes of Health, Bethesda, MD, 1997.

14 Weatherall D J, Ledingham J G G, Warrell D A (eds). Oxford textbook of medicine, 3rd edn. Oxford University Press, Oxford, 1996.

15 Kumar P, Clark M. Clinical medicine, 3rd edn. Baillière Tindall, London, 1994.

16 Rapola J M, Virtamo J, Haukka J K et al. Effect of vitamin E and beta carotene on the incidence of angina pectoris. A randomized, double-blind, controlled trial. JAMA 1996; 275: 693–8.

17 The Alpha-Tocopherol, Beta Carotene Cancer Prevention Study Group. The effect of vitamin E and beta carotene on the incidence of lung cancer and other cancers in male smokers. N Engl J Med 1994; 330: 1029–35.

18 Omenn G S, Goodman G E, Thornquist M D et al. Effects of a combination of beta carotene and vitamin A on lung cancer and cardiovascular disease. N Engl J Med 1996; 334: 1150–5.

19 Haynes R B, Wilczynski N L, McKibbon K A, Walker C J, Sinclair J C. Developing optimal search strategies for detecting clinically sound studies in MEDLINE. J Amer Med Inform Assoc 1994; 1: 447–58.

20 Blakeley D D, Oddone E Z, Hasselblad V, Simel D L, Matchar D B. Noninvasive carotid artery testing. A meta-analytic review. Ann Intern Med 1995; 122: 360–7.

21 Criswell B K, Langsfeld M, Tullis M J, Marek J. Evaluating institutional variability of duplex scanning in the detection of carotid artery stenosis. Am J Surg 1998; 176: 591–7.

22 Bain D J, Fergie N, Quin R O, Greene M. Role of arteriography in the selection of patients for carotid endarterectomy. Br J Surg 1998; 85: 768–70.

23 Sauve J S, Thorpe K E, Sackett D L, Taylor D W, Barnett H J M, Haynes R B, Fox A J, on behalf of the NASCET Investigators. Can bruits distinguish high-grade from moderate symptomatic carotid stenosis? Ann Intern Med 1994; 120: 633–7.

24 Ekbom A, Helmick C, Zack M, Adami H O. Ulcerative colitis and colorectal cancer. A population-based study. N Engl J Med 1990; 323: 1228–33.

25 Lennard-Jones J E, Melville D M, Morson B C et al. Precancer and cancer in extensive ulcerative colitis: findings among 401 patients over 22 years. Gut 1990; 31: 800–6.

26 Palli D, Trallori G, Saieva C, Tarantino O, Edili E, D'Albasio G, Pacini F, Masala G. General and cancer specific mortality of a population based cohort of patients with inflammatory bowel disease: the Florence Study. Gut 1998; 42: 175–9.

27 Stewenius J, Adnerhill I, Anderson H et al. Incidence of colorectal cancer and all cause mortality in non-selected patients with ulcerative colitis and indeterminate colitis in Malmo, Sweden. Int J Colorectal Dis 1995; 10: 117–22.

28 Mellemkjaer L, Olsen J H, Frisch M, Johansen C, Gridley G, McLaughlin J K. Cancer in patients with ulcerative colitis. Int J Cancer 1995; 60: 330–3.

29 Langholz E, Munkholm P, Davidsen M, Binder V. Colorectal cancer risk and mortality in patients with ulcerative colitis. Gastroenterology 1992; 103: 1444–51.

30 Lynch D A, Lobo A J, Sobala G M, Dixon M F, Axon A T. Failure of colonoscopic surveillance in ulcerative colitis. Gut 1993; 34: 1075–83.

31 Shea S, DuMouchel W, Bahamonde L. A meta-analysis of 16 randomized controlled trials to evaluate computer-based clinical reminder systems for preventive care in the ambulatory setting. JAMA 1996; 3(6): 399–409.

32 Review: computerized reminders increase the rate of use of most preventive services. ACP Journal Club 1997; 126: 80. Evidence-Based Medicine 1997 May–June; 2: 96. Abstract of Shea S, DuMouchel W, Bahamonde L A meta-analysis of 16 randomized controlled trials to evaluate computer-based clinical reminder systems for preventive care in the ambulatory setting. J Am Med Inform Assoc 1996; 3: 399–409.

33 Overhage J M, Tierney W M, McDonald C J. Computer reminders to implement preventive care guidelines for hospitalized patients. Arch Intern Med 1996; 156: 1551–6.

Diagnosis and screening

The main part of this chapter has been written to help you answer three questions about diagnostic tests:

1. Is this evidence about the accuracy of a diagnostic test valid?

2. Does this (valid) evidence demonstrate an important ability of this test to accurately distinguish patients who do and don't have a specific disorder?

3. Can I apply this valid, important diagnostic test to a specific patient?

The first two questions, concerning validity and determining importance, are often referred to as "critical appraisal", and can be addressed in either order. Many clinicians (including some of us, some of the time!) prefer to carry out the second step first, because if the report concludes that the impact of a test is unimportant, who cares whether it's valid? The counter approach is to look first at validity, because if the report is invalid, who cares whether it concludes the test is important? We'd suggest that the preferred order depends on their comparative speed and ease, as long as we remember that we have to carry out both steps before going onto the third.

Finally, because the screening and early diagnosis of symptomless individuals have some similarities with, but also some crucial differences from, the diagnosis of sick ones, we'll close with a special section devoted to these acts at the interface of clinical medicine and public health.

IS THIS EVIDENCE ABOUT THE ACCURACY OF A DIAGNOSTIC TEST VALID?

Having found a possibly useful article about a diagnostic test, how can we quickly critically appraise it for its proximity to the truth? This can be done by asking some simple questions, and

Table 3.1 Is this evidence about a diagnostic test valid?

1. Was there an independent, blind comparison with a reference ("gold") standard of diagnosis?

2. Was the diagnostic test evaluated in an appropriate spectrum of patients (like those in whom we would use it in practice)?

3. Was the reference standard applied regardless of the diagnostic test result?

4. Was the test (or cluster of tests) validated in a second, independent group of patients?

often we'll find their answers in the article's abstract. Table 3.1 lists these questions for individual reports, but we can also apply them to the interpretation of a systematic review (overview) of several different studies of the same diagnostic test for the same target disorder.*

1. Was there an independent, blind comparison with a reference ("gold") standard of diagnosis?

This is quite a mouthful, but it simply means that two criteria should have been met. First, the patients in the study should have undergone *both* the diagnostic test in question (say, an item of the history or physical examination, a blood test, etc.) *and* the reference (or "gold") standard (an autopsy or biopsy or other confirmatory "proof" that they do or do not have the target disorder), and second, the results of one should not be known to those who are applying and interpreting the other (e.g. the pathologist interpreting the biopsy that comprises the reference standard for the target disorder should be "blind" to the result of the blood test that comprises the diagnostic test under study). In this way, investigators avoid the conscious and unconscious bias that might otherwise cause the reference standard to be "over-interpreted" when the diagnostic test is positive and "under-interpreted" when it is negative. Sometimes investigators have a difficult time coming up with clear-cut

---

* As we'll stress throughout this book, systematic reviews provide us with the most valid and useful external evidence on just about any clinical question we can pose. They are still pretty rare for diagnostic tests, and for this reason we'll describe them in their usual, therapeutic habitat, in Chapter 5. When applying Table 5.9 to diagnostic tests, simply substitute "diagnostic test" for "treatment" as you read.

reference standards (e.g. for psychiatric disorders), and we'll want to give careful consideration to their arguments justifying the selection of their reference standard. Moreover, we caution you against the uncritical acceptance of reference standards, even when they are based on "expert" interpretations of biopsies; in a recent *Evidence-Based Medicine* note, Kenneth Fleming[1] reported that the degree of agreement over and above chance in reading breast, skin and liver biopsies is less than 50%!

One way or another, the report will wind up calling some results "normal" and others "abnormal", and we'll show you how to interpret these in the next section of this chapter. For now, you might simply want to recognize that there are six definitions of "normal" in common use (listed in Table 3.2). This chapter will use definition #5 ("diagnostic" normal) because we think that the first four are flawed. The first two (the Gaussian and percentile definitions) focus just on the diagnostic test results, with no reference standard, and define the "normal range" on the basis of statistical properties (standard deviations or percentiles). They not only imply that all "abnormalities" occur at the same frequency, but suggest that if we perform more and more diagnostic tests on our patient, we are increasingly likely to find something "abnormal", thus leading to all sorts of inappropriate further testing.

Table 3.2 Six definitions of normal

1. **Gaussian**: the mean ± 2 standard deviations – this one assumes a normal distribution for all tests and results in all "abnormalities" having the same frequency.

2. **Percentile**: within the range, say of 5–95% – has the same basic defect as the Gaussian definition.

3. **Culturally desirable**: when "normal" is that which is preferred by society, the role of medicine gets confused.

4. **Risk factor**: carrying no additional risk of disease; nicely labels the outliers, but does changing a risk factor necessarily change risk?

5. **Diagnostic**: range of results beyond which target disorders become highly probable; the focus of this discussion.

6. **Therapeutic**: range of results beyond which treatment does more good than harm; means we have to keep up with advances in therapy!

The third definition of "normal" (culturally desirable) represents the sorts of value judgement seen in fashion advertisements, and at the fringes of the "lifestyle" movement where medicine becomes confused with morality. The fourth (risk factor) definition has the drawback that it "labels" or stigmatizes some patients regardless of whether we can intervene to lower their risk, a big problem with neonatal genetic testing and other screening maneuvers, as you'll learn in the concluding section of this chapter. The fifth (diagnostic) definition is the one that we will focus on here, and we will show you how to work with it in the next bit of this chapter. The final (therapeutic) definition (does treating at and beyond this level do more good than harm?) is in part an outgrowth of the fourth (risk factor) definition, but has the great clinical advantage that it changes with our knowledge of efficacy. Thus, the definition of normal blood pressure has changed radically over the past few decades as we have learned that treatment of progressively less pronounced elevations of blood pressure does more good than harm.

2. Was the diagnostic test evaluated in an appropriate spectrum of patients (like those in whom we would use it in practice)?

Did the report include patients possessing all the common presentations of the target disorder (including those with its early manifestations), and patients with other, commonly confused diagnoses? Studies that confine themselves to florid cases vs. asymptomatic volunteers are not very informative, for when the diagnosis is obvious to the eye we don't need any diagnostic test. The really useful articles are the ones in which the diagnostic test was applied to patients with mild as well as severe, and early as well as late cases of the target disorder, and among both treated and untreated individuals. In addition, we would want the diagnostic test to have been applied to patients with different disorders that are commonly confused with the target disorder of interest.

3. Was the reference standard applied regardless of the diagnostic test result?

When patients have a negative diagnostic test result, investigators are tempted to forego applying the reference standard, and when the latter is invasive or risky (e.g. angiography) it may be wrong to carry it out on patients with negative test results. To overcome this, many investigators now employ a reference standard for proving that a patient does not have the target disorder which requires that the patient doesn't suffer any adverse health outcome during a long follow-up despite the absence of any definitive treatment (e.g. convincing evidence that a patient with clinically suspected deep vein thrombosis did not have this disorder would include no ill-effects during a prolonged follow-up despite the absence of anti-thrombotic therapy).

4. Was the test (or cluster of tests) validated in a second, independent group of patients?

Diagnostic tests are predictors, not explainers, of diagnoses. As a result, their initial evaluation cannot distinguish between real diagnostic accuracy for the target disorder and chance associations due to idiosyncrasies in the initial ("training" or "derivation") set of patients. This problem is compounded for clusters of diagnostic features (often called "clinical prediction guides"). The best indicator of accuracy in these situations is the demonstration of similar levels of accuracy when the test or cluster is evaluated in a second, independent (or "test") set of patients. If it performs well in this "test" set, we are reassured about its accuracy. If it performs poorly, we should look elsewhere. And if no "test set" study has been carried out, we'd be wise to reserve judgement. We'll meet clinical prediction guides again in the next chapter when they are used to make prognoses.

If the report we're reading fails one or more of these four tests, we'll need to consider whether it has a fatal flaw that renders its conclusions invalid; if so, it's back to more searching (either now or later; if we've already used up our time for this week, perhaps we can interest a colleague or trainee in taking this on as an "educational prescription" – see p. 24 if this term is new to you). On the other hand, if the report passes this initial scrutiny and we decide that we can believe its results, and we haven't already carried out the second critical appraisal step of deciding whether these results are important, then we can proceed to the next section.

DOES THIS (VALID) EVIDENCE DEMONSTRATE AN IMPORTANT ABILITY OF THIS TEST TO ACCURATELY DISTINGUISH PATIENTS WHO DO AND DON'T HAVE A SPECIFIC DISORDER?

Sensitivity, specificity, and likelihood ratios

In deciding whether the evidence about a diagnostic test is important, we will focus on the accuracy of the test in distinguishing patients with and without the target disorder, in terms of both the old-fashioned concepts of sensitivity and specificity and the new-fangled and more powerful ideas around likelihood ratios. What we will focus on here is the ability of a valid test to change our minds from what we thought before the test (we'll call that the "pre-test" probability of some target disorder) to what we think afterward (we'll call that the "post-test" probability of the target disorder). Diagnostic tests that produce big changes from pre-test to post-test probabilities are important and likely to be useful to us in our practice.

Suppose that we're working up a patient with anemia and think that the probability that she has iron deficiency anemia is 50%, i.e. the odds are about 50:50 that it's due to iron deficiency. When we present the patient to our boss, we ask for an educational prescription to determine the usefulness of performing a serum ferritin on our patient as a means of detecting iron deficiency anemia. Suppose further that, in filling our prescription we find a systematic review of several studies of this diagnostic test (evaluated against the reference standard of a bone marrow stain for iron), decide that it is valid (based on the guides in Table 3.1), and find their results as shown in Table 3.3. By the time we've tracked down and studied the external evidence, our patient's serum ferritin comes back at 60 mmol/L. How should we put all this together?

As you can see from Table 3.3, our patient's result (60 mmol/L) places her in the top row of the table, either in cell a or cell b. From that fact you might notice several things. First, you might note that 90% of patients with iron deficiency have serum ferritins in the same range as our patient [a/(a + c)]; that property, the proportion of patients with the target disorder who have positive test results, is called "sensitivity". And you might also note that only 15% of patients with other causes

Table 3.3 Results of a systematic review of serum ferritin as a diagnostic test for iron deficiency anemia[a]

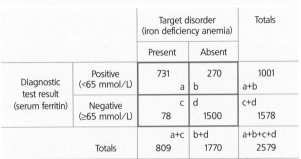

		Target disorder (iron deficiency anemia)		Totals
		Present	Absent	
Diagnostic test result (serum ferritin)	Positive (<65 mmol/L)	731 a	270 b	1001 $a+b$
	Negative (≥65 mmol/L)	c 78	d 1500	$c+d$ 1578
	Totals	$a+c$ 809	$b+d$ 1770	$a+b+c+d$ 2579

[a] These data come from: Guyatt G H, Oxman A D, Ali M, Willan A, Malloy W, Patterson C. Laboratory diagnosis of iron-deficiency anemia: an overview. J Gen Intern Med 1992; 7: 145−53.

Sensitivity = $a/(a + c)$ = 731/809 = 90%.

Specificity = $d/(b + d)$ = 1500/1770 = 85%.

LR + = sens/(1 − spec) = 90%/15% = 6.

LR − = (1 − sens)/spec = 10%/85% = 0.12.

Positive predictive value = $a/(a + b)$ = 731/1001 = 73%.

Negative predictive value = $d/(c + d)$ = 1500/1578 = 95%.

Prevalence = $(a + c)/(a + b + c + d)$ = 809/2579 = 31%.

Pre-test odds = prevalence/(1 − prevalence) = 31%/69% = 0.45.

Post-test odds = pre-test odds × likelihood ratio.

Post-test probability = post-test odds/(post-test odds + 1).

of their anemia have results in the same range as our patient,[†] which means that our patient's result would be about six times as likely (90%/15%) to be seen in someone with iron deficiency anemia than in someone without the condition; that ratio is called the "likelihood ratio" for a positive test result (LR+) and another way of thinking about (and calculating) it is to divide sensitivity by (1 − specificity). Third, since we'd

---

[†] The complement of this proportion describes the proportion of patients who do not have the target disorder who have negative or normal test results, d/(c+d), and is called specificity.

thought ahead of time (before we had the result of the serum ferritin) that our patient's odds of iron deficiency were 50:50, that's called a pre-test odds of 1:1. Fourth, as you can see from the formulae towards the bottom of Table 3.3, we can multiply that pre-test odds of 1 by the likelihood ratio of 6 to get the post-test odds of iron deficiency anemia after the test ($1 \times 6 = 6$); that's a post-test odds of 6:1 in favor of iron deficiency anemia. Since, like most clinicians, you may be more comfortable thinking in terms of probabilities than odds, this post-test odds of 6:1 converts (as you can see at the bottom of Table 3.3) to a post-test probability of $6/(6+1) = 6/7 = 86\%$. So, it looks like we've made the diagnosis, and this diagnostic test has generated an important result for our patient. (To check yourself out on these calculations, try calculating the post-test probability for the same ferritin result for a patient who, like those in Table 3.3, has a pre-test odds of 0.47;[‡] you'll know you did it right if you wind up with an answer for post-test probability that is identical to its equivalent, the positive predictive value.)

Extremely high values of sensitivity and specificity are useful, but not for the reasons you may think.[§] When a test has a very high sensitivity (such as the loss of retinal vein pulsation in increased intracranial pressure), a negative result (the presence of pulsation) effectively rules out the diagnosis (of raised intracranial pressure), and one of our clinical clerks suggested that we apply the mnemonic "SnNout" to such findings (when a sign has a high **Sen**sitivity, a **N**egative result rules **out** the diagnosis). Similarly, when a sign has a very high **Sp**ecificity (such as the face of a child with Down's syndrome), a **P**ositive result effectively rules **in** the diagnosis (of Down's); not surprisingly, our clinical clerks call such a finding a "SpPin". We've listed some SpPins and SnNouts in Table 3.4, and have generated a longer list on our website <http://www.library.utoronto.ca/medicine/ebm/>.

[‡] The post-test odds are $0.45 \times 6 = 2.7$ and the post-test probability is $2.7/3.7 = 73\%$. Note that this is identical to the positive predictive value.

[§] On first encounter, many learners think that tests with high sensitivity are useful for "ruling in" diagnoses and tests with high specificity are useful for "ruling them out"; in fact, the reverse is the case.

Table 3.4 Some SpPins and SnNouts[a]

Target disorder	SpPin (and specificity) [presence rules in the target disorder]	SnNout (and sensitivity) [absence rules out the target disorder]
Ascites (by imaging or tap)[b]	Fluid wave (92%)	History of ankle swelling (93%)
Pleural effusion[c]	Auscultatory percussion note loud and sharp (100%)	Auscultatory percussion note soft and/or dull (96%)
Increased intracranial pressure (by CAT scan or direct measurement)[d]		Loss of spontaneous retinal vein pulsation (100%)
Cancer as a cause of lower back pain (by further investigation)[e]		Age > 50 or cancer history or unexplained weight loss or failure of conservative therapy (100%)
Sinusitis (by further investigation)[f]		Maxillary toothache or purulent nasal secretion or poor response to nasal decongestants or abnormal transillumination or history of colored nasal discharge (LR = 0.1)
Alcohol abuse or dependency[g]	Yes to >3 of the CAGE questions (99.8%)	
Splenomegaly (by imaging)[h]	Positive percussion (Nixon method) and palpation	
Non-urgent cause for dizziness[i]	Positive head-hanging test and either vertigo or vomiting (94%)	

[a] To find more examples, and to nominate additions to the databank of SpPins and SnNouts, refer to this textbook's website at: <http://www.library.utoronto.ca/medicine/ebm/>.

[b] JAMA 1992; 267: 2645–8.
[c] J Gen Int Med 1994; 9: 71–4.
[d] Arch Neurol 1978; 35: 37–40.
[e] JAMA 1992; 268: 760–5.
[f] JAMA 1993; 270: 1242–6.
[g] Am J Med 1987; 82: 231–5.
[h] JAMA 1993; 270: 2218–21.
[i] JAMA 1994; 271: 385–8.

Multilevel likelihood ratios

Although the serum ferritin determination looks impressive when viewed in terms of its sensitivity (90%) and specificity (85%), the newer way of expressing its accuracy with likelihood ratios reveals its even greater power and, in this particular example, shows how we can be misled by the old sensitivity–specificity approach that restricts us to just two levels (positive and negative) of the test result. Most test results, like serum ferritin, can be divided into several levels, and in Table 3.5 we show you a particularly useful way of dividing test results into five levels.

When this is done, we see how much information about ferritin's accuracy we lost when we confined the test results to just "positive" or "negative". The LR for the "very positive" result is a huge 52, so that one extreme level of the test result can be shown to rule in the diagnosis, and in this case we can SpPin 59% (474/809) of the patients with iron deficiency anemia, despite the unimpressive sensitivity (59%) that would have been achieved if the ferritin results had been split just below this level. Likelihood ratios of 10 or more, when applied to pre-test probabilities of 33% or more (0.33/0.67 = pre-test odds of 0.5) will generate post-test probabilities of 5/6 = 83% or more.

Moreover, the other extreme level (<95) can SnNout 75% (1332/1770) of those who do not have iron deficiency anemia (again despite a not-very-impressive specificity of 75%). Likelihood ratios of 0.1 or less, when applied to pre-test probabilities of 33% or less (0.33/0.67 = pre-test odds of 0.5) will generate post-test probabilities of 0.05/1.05 = 5% or less. The two intermediate levels (moderately positive and moderately negative) can move a 50% prior probability (pre-test odds of 1:1) to the useful but not necessarily diagnostic post-test probabilities of 4.8/5.8 = 83% and 0.39/1.39 = 28%. And the indeterminate level ("neutral") in the middle (containing about 10% of both sorts of patients) can be seen to be uninformative, with a likelihood ratio of 1. When diagnostic test results are around 1.0, we've learned nothing by ordering them. To give you a better "feel" for this, the impact of different likelihood ratios on different pre-test

Table 3.5 The usefulness of five levels of a diagnostic test result

Diagnostic test result	Target disorder (Iron deficiency) present		Target disorder absent		Likelihood ratio	Diagnostic impact
Serum ferritin (mmol/L)	Number	%	Number	%		
Very positive	< 15	474	59 (474/809)	20	1.1 (20/1770)	52	Rule-in "SpPin"
Moderately positive	15–34	175	22 (175/809)	79	4.5 (79/1770)	4.8	Intermediate high
Neutral	35–64	82	10 (82/809)	171	10 (171/1770)	1	Indeterminate
Moderately negative	65–94	30	3.7 (30/809)	168	9.5 (168/1770)	0.39	Intermediate low
Extremely negative	≥ 95	48	5.9 (48/809)	1332	75 (1332/1770)	0.08	Rule-out "SnNout"
		809	100 (809/809)	1770	100 (1770/1770)		

Table 3.6 Some post-test probabilities generated by five levels of a diagnostic test result

Likelihood ratio	Post-test probability of the target disorder for different pre-test probabilities					
	Pre-test 5%	Pre-test 10%	Pre-test 20%	Pre-test 30%	Pre-test 50%	Pre-test 70%
Very positive 10	34%	53%	71%	81%	91%	96%
Moderately positive 3	14%	25%	43%	56%	75%	88%
Neutral 1	5%	10%	20%	30%	50%	70%
Moderately negative 0.3	1.5%	3.2%	7%	11%	23%	41%
Extremely negative 0.1	0.5%	1%	2.5%	4%	9%	19%

probabilities are shown in Table 3.6. We've provided additional examples of likelihood ratios on this book's website: <http://www.library.utoronto.ca/medicine/ebm/>.

Finally, there's an easier way of manipulating all these probability ↔ odds calculations, and a nomogram for doing so appears as Figure 3.1 and in the pocket cards that come with this book. You can check out your understanding of this nomogram by using it to replicate the results of Tables 3.5 and 3.6.

Now return to our patient with a pre-test probability for iron deficiency of 50% and a ferritin result of 60 mmol/L. To your surprise (we reckon!), our patient's test result generates an indeterminate likelihood ratio of only 1, and the test which we thought might be very useful, based on the old sensitivity and specificity way of looking at things, really hasn't been helpful in moving us toward the diagnosis. We'll have to think about other tests (including perhaps the reference standard of a bone marrow examination) to sort out her diagnosis.

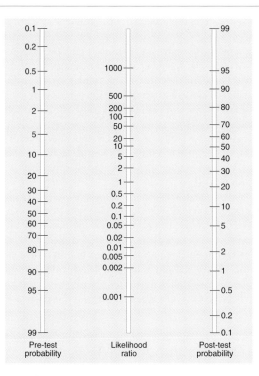

Figure 3.1 A likelihood ratio nomogram.

More and more reports of diagnostic tests are providing multilevel likelihood ratios as measures of their accuracy. When their abstracts report only sensitivity and specificity, we can sometimes find a table with more levels and generate our own set of likelihood ratios; at other times we can find a scatterplot (of test results vs. diagnoses) that is good enough for us to be able to split them into levels. Even if all we have is sensitivity and specificity, we can generate likelihood ratios from them by reference to the formulae in Table 3.3 (the likelihood ratio for a positive test result = LR+ = sensitivity/[1 − specificity] and the likelihood ratio for a negative test result = LR− = [1 − sensitivity]/specificity).

Some reports into the accuracy of diagnostic tests go beyond even likelihood ratios, and one of their extensions deserves mention here. This extension considers multiple diagnostic tests as a cluster or sequence of tests for a given target disorder. These multiple results can be presented in different ways, either as clusters of positive/negative results or as multivariate scores, and in either case they can be ranked and handled just like other multilevel likelihood ratios. When they perform (nearly) as well in a second, independent ("test") set of patients, we often refer to them as "clinical prediction guides" (CPGs). We'll encounter such CPGs again in the chapter on prognosis (Ch. 4).

In any event, having decided that a diagnostic test is both valid and accurate, we can now move to the final issue of how to integrate the results of this critical appraisal with our patient's unique pre-test probability and our individual clinical expertise. However, if you jumped to this second consideration of importance without first determining whether the evidence about this diagnostic test was valid, you'd better go back before you go forward!

CAN I APPLY THIS VALID, IMPORTANT DIAGNOSTIC TEST TO A SPECIFIC PATIENT?

Having found a valid systematic review or individual report about a diagnostic test, and having decided that its accuracy is sufficiently high that it would be useful, how do we integrate it with our patient's unique pre-test probability and apply it to our patient? There are three questions whose answers dictate this determination, and they are summarized in Table 3.7.

1. Is the diagnostic test available, affordable, accurate, and precise in our setting?

This is the first question we need to answer. We obviously can't order a test that is not available, but even if it is, we may want to check around to be sure that it's performed and interpreted in a competent, reproducible fashion and that its potential consequences (see below) justify its cost. Moreover, diagnostic tests often behave differently among different

Table 3.7 Questions to answer in applying a valid diagnostic test to an individual patient

1. Is the diagnostic test available, affordable, accurate, and precise in our setting?

2. Can we generate a clinically sensible estimate of our patient's pre-test probability?
   - From personal experience, prevalence statistics, practice databases, or primary studies
   - Are the study patients similar to our own?
   - Is it unlikely that the disease possibilities or probabilities have changed since this evidence was gathered?

3. Will the resulting post-test probabilities affect our management and help our patient?
   - Could it move us across a test-treatment threshold?
   - Would our patient be a willing partner in carrying it out?
   - Would the consequences of the test help our patient reach his or her goals in all this?

subsets of patients, generating higher likelihood ratios in later stages of florid disease, and lower likelihood ratios in early, mild stages. This is another reason why multilevel likelihood ratios are helpful, as there are at least theoretical reasons why they should suffer less distortion from this cause.

Finally, at least some diagnostic tests based on symptoms or signs lose power as patients move from primary care to secondary and tertiary care. Reference back to Table 3.3 can show you why. If patients are referred onward, in part because of symptoms, their primary care clinicians will be sending along patients in both cells a and b, and subsequent evaluations of the accuracy of their symptoms will tend to show falling specificity due to the referral of patients with false-positive findings. If we think that any of these factors may be operating, we can try out what we judge to be clinically sensible variations in the likelihood ratios for the test result and see whether the results alter our post-test probabilities in a way that changes our diagnosis (the short-hand term for this sort of exploration is "sensitivity analysis").

2. Can we generate a clinically sensible estimate of our patient's pre-test probability?

This is a key topic, and deserves its own "section-within-a-section". How can we estimate our patient's pre-test probability? We've used five different sources for this vital information: clinical experience, regional or national prevalence statistics, practice databases, the original report we used for deciding on the accuracy and importance of the test, and studies devoted specifically to determining pre-test probabilities. We'll take these in turn.

First, we can recall our clinical experience with prior patients who presented with the same clinical problem, and back-track from their final diagnoses to their pre-test probabilities. While easily and quickly accessed, our memories are often distorted by our last patient, our most dramatic (or embarrassing) patient, our fear of missing a rare but treatable cause, and the like, so we use this source with caution.** And if we're at the beginning of our careers, we may not have enough clinical experience to draw upon. Thus, while we always use our remembered cases, we need to learn to supplement them with other sources, unless we have the time and energy to document all of our diagnoses and generate our own database (see source #3 below).

Second, we could turn to regional or national prevalence statistics on the frequencies of the target disorders in the general population or some subset of it. Estimates from these sources are only as good as the accuracy of their diagnoses, and although they can provide some guidance for "baseline" pre-test probabilities before taking symptoms into account (useful, say, for patients walking into a general practice), even GPs may be more interested in pre-test probabilities in just those persons with a particular symptom.

Third, we could overcome the foregoing problems by tracking down local, regional or national practice databases that collect

---

** If you want to read more about how our minds and memories can distort our clinical reasoning, start with: Kassirer J P, Kopelman R I. Cognitive errors in diagnosis: instantiation, classification, and consequences. Am J Med 1989; 86: 433–441.

patients with the same clinical problem and report the frequency of disorders diagnosed in these patients. While some examples exist, such databases are mostly things of the future. As before, their usefulness will depend on the extent to which they use sensible diagnostic criteria and clear definitions of presenting symptoms.

Fourth, we could simply apply the pre-test probabilities observed in the study we critically appraised for the accuracy and importance of the diagnostic test. If they really did sample the full spectrum of patients with the symptom or clinical problem (the second of our accuracy guides), we can extrapolate the pre-test probability from their study patients (or some subgroup of it) to our patient.

Fifth and finally, we could track down a research report of a study expressly devoted to documenting pre-test probabilities for the array of diagnoses that present with a specific set of symptoms and signs similar to our patient. When done well, among patients closely similar to our patient, these studies provide the least biased source of pre-test probabilities for our use. Such studies are challenging to carry out, and one of us led the group who generated guides for their critical appraisal.[2] We've summarized these guides in Table 3.8.

Table 3.8 Guides for critically appraising a report about pre-test probabilities of disease

1. Is this evidence about pre-test probability valid?
   - Did the study patients represent the full spectrum of those who present with this clinical problem?
   - Were the criteria for each final diagnosis explicit and credible?
   - Was the diagnostic work-up comprehensive and consistently applied?
   - For initially undiagnosed patients, was follow-up sufficiently long and complete?

2. Is this evidence about pre-test probability important?
   - What were the diagnoses and their probabilities?
   - How precise were these estimates of disease probability?

You'll see that most of them are already familiar to you, for they apply equally to reports of the accuracy and importance of diagnostic tests.

We've provided examples of pre-test probabilities in Table 3.9 and will add to this list from our website: <http://www.library.utoronto.ca/medicine/ebm/>.

3. Will the resulting post-test probabilities affect our management and help our patient?

The elements of the answer to this final question are three and begin with the bottom line: could its results move us across some threshold that would cause us to stop all further testing? Two thresholds should be borne in mind, as shown in Figure 3.2.

First, if the diagnostic test was negative or generated a likelihood ratio down near 0.1, the post-test probability might become so low that we would abandon the diagnosis we were pursuing, and turn to other diagnostic possibilities. Put in terms of thresholds, this negative test result has moved us from above to below the "test threshold" in Figure 3.2 and we won't do any more tests for that diagnostic possibility. On the other hand, if the diagnostic test came back positive or generated a high likelihood ratio, the post-test probability might become so high that we would also abandon further testing because we'd made our diagnosis and would now move to choosing the

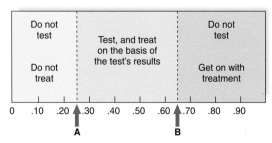

Figure 3.2 Test–treatment thresholds.

Table 3.9 Examples of pre-test probabilities

Symptom or clinical problem	Source	Work-up	Disease probabilities
Anemia of chronic disease	90 adults admitted to a general medical ward of a county hospital in North America[a]	Clinical exam, blood testing, selected other testing	Infection, 36% Inflammation, 6% Malignant, 19% Renal, 15% Other, 24%
Dizziness > 2 weeks	100 adult patients seen in primary care sites in one North American city[b]	Clinical exam, neurological, ophthalmologic, and psychological testing, selected other tests	Vertigo, 54% Psychiatric, 16% Multicausal, 13% Other, 19% Unknown, 8%
Dyspnea > 4 weeks, unexplained by exam, radiograph and spirometry	72 adults referred to outpatient pulmonary clinic in North America[c]	Standardized exam, testing and treatment	Respiratory, 36% Cardiac, 14% Hyperventilation, 19% Other, 12% Unexplained, 19%
Epilepsy, new onset in adults	333 adults presenting to a major urban emergency department in North America (excluded alcohol, head trauma, hypoglycemia)[d]	Standardized exam, testing (including head CT), and treatment	Unknown, 44% Stroke, 11% Tumor, 7% Infection, 17% Metabolic, 5% Other, 16%
Palpitations	190 patients from acute care sites in one North American city[e]	Clinical exam, cardiac and psychological testing, selected other tests	Cardiac, 43% Psychiatric, 31% Miscellaneous, 10% Unknown, 16%
Raynaud's phenomenon	Literature review of published reports of secondary diseases in 639 patients with Raynaud's, from various settings[f]	Variable, usually clinical exam, selected serology and follow-up	Only 12.6% had or developed "secondary" disorders (e.g. systemic sclerosis, MCTD, SLE, etc.)

[a] Am J Med 1989; 87: 638–44. [b] Ann Intern Med 1992; 117: 898–904.
[c] Chest 1991; 100: 1293–9. [d] Ann Emerg Med 1994; 24: 1108–14.
[e] Am J Med 1996; 100: 138–48. [f] Arch Intern Med 1998; 158: 595–600.

most appropriate therapy; in these terms, we've now crossed from below to above the "treatment threshold" in Figure 3.2. It is only if our diagnostic test result leaves us stranded between the test and treatment thresholds that we would continue to pursue that initial diagnosis by performing other tests. Although there are some very fancy ways of calculating test–treatment thresholds from test accuracy and the risks and benefits of correct and incorrect diagnostic conclusions,[††] intuitive test–treatment thresholds are commonly used by experienced clinicians and are another example of individual clinical expertise.

We may not cross a test–treatment threshold until we've performed several different diagnostic tests, and here is where another nice property of the likelihood ratio comes into play. Because the post-test odds for the first diagnostic test we apply is the pre-test odds for our second diagnostic test, we needn't switch back and forth between odds and probabilities between tests. We can simply keep multiplying the running product by the likelihood ratio generated from the next test. For example, when a 45-year-old man walks into our office, his pre-test probability of >75% stenosis of one or more of his coronary arteries is about 6%. Suppose that he gives us a history of atypical chest pain (only two of the three symptoms of substernal chest discomfort, brought on by exertion, and relieved in less than 10 minutes by rest are present, generating a likelihood ratio of about 13) and that his exercise ECG reveals 2.2 mm of non-sloping ST-segment depression (generating a likelihood ratio of about 11). Then his post-test probability for coronary stenosis is his pre-test probability (converted into odds) times the product of the likelihood ratios generated from his history (13) and exercise ECG (11), with the resulting post-test odds converted back to probabilities (through dividing by its value + 1), i.e.:

$$(0.06/0.94) \times 13 \times 11 = 9.13, \text{ and then } 9.13/10.13 = 90\%$$

The final result of these calculations is strictly accurate as long as the diagnostic tests being combined are "independent"

[††] See the recommendations for additional reading or: Pauker S G, Kassirer J P. The threshold approach to clinical decision making. N Engl J Med 1980; 302: 1109.

(i.e. the probability of a specific result on the second is the same for every result on the first), and we know intuitively that this is not true for most of the diagnostic tests we apply in sequences aiming toward a single diagnosis. Accordingly, we would want the calculated post-test probability at the end of this sequence to be comfortably above our treatment threshold before we would act upon it. This additional example of how likelihood ratios make lots of implicit diagnostic reasoning explicit is another argument in favor of seeking reports of overall likelihood ratios for sequences or clusters of diagnostic tests.

We should have kept our patient informed as we worked our way through all the foregoing considerations, especially if we've concluded that the diagnostic test is worth considering. If we haven't yet done so, we certainly need to do so now. Every diagnostic test involves some invasion of privacy, and some are embarrassing, painful, or dangerous. We'll have to be sure that the patient is an informed, willing partner in the undertaking.

Finally, the ultimate question to ask about using any diagnostic test is whether its consequences (reassurance when negative, labeling and possibly generating awful diagnostic and prognostic news if positive, leading to further diagnostic tests and treatments, etc.) will help our patient achieve his or her goals of therapy. Included here are considerations of how subsequent interventions match clinical guidelines or restrictions on access to therapy designed to optimize the use of finite resources for all members of our society.

LEARNING AND TEACHING WITH CATS

Now that we have invested precious time and energy into finding and critically appraising an article, it would be a shame not to summarize and keep track of it so that we (and others) can use it again in the future. The means that Stephane Sauve, Hui Lee, and Mike Farkouh, residents on Dave Sackett's clinical service a few years ago, invented to accomplish this was to create a standardized one-page summary of the evidence organized as a "critically appraised topic", which they called a "CAT". A CAT begins with a declarative title and quickly states a clinical "bottom line" describing the clinical action that follows from the paper. To assist later updating of the CAT, the three- or four-part clinical question that started the process, and the search terms that were used to locate the paper are included in it. Next is a summary of the study methods and a table summarizing the key results. Any issues important to bear in mind when applying the CAT (such as rare adverse effects, costs, or unusual elements of the critical appraisal) are inserted beneath the results table.

EBM teachers routinely suggest to their learners that they create CATs when they are filling their educational prescriptions (see Ch. 1). This process both reinforces the critical appraisal process and creates an extremely valuable ongoing educational resource for the clinical team. To help generate CATs, we've placed a CATnipper version (with nine lives) that can be downloaded from the book's website: <http://www.library.utoronto.ca/medicine/ebm/>. This software takes learners step by step through the creation of a CAT, calculates some of the clinically useful measures of therapy (NNTs, likelihood ratios) and automatically generates their confidence intervals. The CATMaker allows CATs to be saved (even in a draft "kitten" form that can be retrieved for later revision) or outputted in ".txt" files or ".html" formats. This means that you can create your own database to store your CATs in an easily retrievable format, make copies available to your students and colleagues, or even place them on your local intranet. Now take a look at the CAT we generated for ferritin.

SCREENING AND CASE-FINDING

The previous bits of this chapter have focussed on making a diagnosis among sick patients who have come to us for help. They are asking us to diagnose their ills and to help them as best we can, and only charlatans guarantee them longer life at the initial encounter. This final bit of the chapter turns the tables and focuses on making early diagnoses of pre-symptomatic disease among well individuals in the general public (we'll call that "screening") or among patients who have come to us for some other unrelated disorder

CAT Ferritin can diagnose iron deficiency in the elderly

Clinical bottom line Serum ferritin can be very useful in diagnosing iron deficiency anemia in the elderly.

Clinical scenario. 75 y/o retired schoolteacher (in for a check-up) found to have a Hb of 10, with an MCV of 80, a negative history and physical, and no meds likely to suppress her marrow or cause a bleed. I think her probability of iron deficiency is 1 out of 2 or 50%.

Three-part question. In an elderly symptomless woman with mild anemia, would a serum ferritin help determine whether her bone marrow iron stores were depleted?

Search terms. In Best Evidence, I searched on "ferritin" and got six hits (plus normal values), including a great single study and an overview.

Appraised by: Sackett in the CEBM, Oxford; Friday, July 09, 1999

The study

Independent ... ?	Yes
Blind ... ?	Yes
Standard applied regardless of test result ... ?	Yes
Appropriate spectrum ... ?	Can't tell

Target disorder and gold standard. Bone marrow, stained for iron.

Patients. Consecutive anemic patients in several in-patient and outpatient settings. Transfused patients excluded.

Diagnostic test. Serum ferritin by radioimmunoassay.

The evidence

	Present		Absent		
Test result	No.	Prop.	No.	Prop.	LR
< 15	474	0.59	20	0.01	51.85
15–34	175	0.22	79	0.04	4.85
35–64	82	0.10	171	0.11	1.05
65–94	30	0.04	168	0.09	0.39
≥ 95	48	0.06	1332	0.75	0.08

Comments

1. For elderly patients with symptomless anemia, go to the CAT on anemia in the elderly to determine the yields from upper and lower GI investigations.
2. Lots of labs are very slow in returning ferritin requests.

Expiry date: Jan 2001.

References

Guyatt G H, Oxman A D, Ali M et al. Laboratory diagnosis of iron deficiency anemia: an overview. J Gen Intern Med 1992; 7: 45–53.

Patterson C, Guyatt G H, Singer J, Ali M, Turpie I. Iron deficiency in the elderly: the diagnostic process. Can Med Assoc J 1991; 144: 435–40.

(we'll call that "case-finding"). Individuals undergoing screening and case-finding are *not* ill from the target disorders, and we are soliciting them with the guarantee (overt or covert) that they will live longer, or at least better, if they let us test them. Accordingly, the evidence we need about the validity of screening and case-finding goes beyond the accuracy of the test for early diagnosis; we need hard evidence that patients are better off, in the long run, when such early diagnosis is achieved.

This is because all screening and case-finding, at least in the short-run, hurt people. Early diagnosis is just that: people are "labeled" as having, or as being at high risk for developing, some pretty awful diseases (cancer of the breast, stroke, heart attack, and the like). And this labeling takes place months, years, or even decades before the awful diseases will become manifest as symptomatic illness (often in only a small portion of those who screen positive). Labeling hurts. For example, a cohort of working men studied both before and after they were labeled hypertensive displayed increased absenteeism, decreased psychological well-being, and progressive loss of income in comparison to their normotensive workmates (and these bad effects could not be blamed on drug side-effects, for they occurred even among men who were never treated!).[3] What's even worse is that those with false-positive screening tests will experience only harm (regardless of the efficacy of early treatment). But even individuals with true-positive tests who receive efficacious treatment have had "healthy time" taken away from them; early diagnosis may not make folks live longer, but it surely makes all of them "sick" longer!

We've placed this discussion at the end of the chapter on diagnosis, with the chapter on therapy the next but one, on purpose. In order to decide whether screening and case-finding do more good than harm, we'll have to consider the validity of claims about both the accuracy of the early diagnostic test and the efficacy of the therapy that follows it. We've summarized the guides for doing this in Table 3.10. Its elements are discussed in greater detail elsewhere (consult the "Further reading" at the end of this chapter).

Table 3.10 Guides for deciding whether a screening or early diagnostic maneuver does more good than harm

1. Does early diagnosis really lead to improved survival, or quality of life, or both?
2. Are the early diagnosed patients willing partners in the treatment strategy?
3. Is the time and energy it will take us to confirm the diagnosis and provide (lifelong) care well spent?
4. Do the frequency and severity of the target disorder warrant this degree of effort and expenditure?

1. Does early diagnosis really lead to improved survival, or quality of life, or both?

Follow-up studies of placebo groups in RCTs have taught us that patients who faithfully follow health advice (by volunteering for screening or by taking their medicine) are destined for better outcomes before they begin, and early diagnostic maneuvers preferentially identify patients with slower progressing, more benign disease. As a result, the only evidence we can trust in determining whether early diagnosis does more good than harm is a true experiment in which individuals were randomly assigned to undergo the early detection test (and, if truly positive, treated for the target disorder) or to be left alone (and only treated if and when they developed symptomatic disease). It was evidence of this sort that showed the benefit of breast examinations and mammography for reducing deaths from breast cancer,[‡‡] and showed the uselessness (indeed, harm) of chest X-rays for lung cancer. Ideally, their follow-up will consider functional and quality-of-life outcomes as well as mortality and discrete clinical events, and we should not be satisfied when the only favorable changes are confined to "risk factors".

2. Are the early diagnosed patients willing partners in the treatment strategy?

Even when therapy is efficacious, patients who refuse or forget to take it cannot benefit from it and are left with only the

---

[‡‡] Because only about a third of women whose breast cancers are diagnosed early go on to prolonged survival, even in this case the majority of positive screenees are harmed, not helped, by early detection.

damage produced by labeling. Early diagnosis will do more harm than good to these patients, and we forget the magnitude of this problem at their peril (even by self-report, only half of patients describe themselves as "compliant"). There are quick ways of diagnosing low compliance and we'll show them to you in Chapter 5 (they comprise looking for non-attendance and non-responsiveness, and by non-confrontational questioning), but this is a diagnosis that you need to establish before, not after, you carry out any screening or case-finding.

3. Is the time and energy it will take us to confirm the diagnosis and provide (lifelong) care well spent?

4. Do the frequency and severity of the target disorder warrant this degree of effort and expenditure?

These questions raise, at the levels of both our individual practice and our community, the unavoidable question of rationing. Is going after the early diagnosis of this condition worth sacrificing the other good we could accomplish by devoting our own or our town's resources to some other purpose?

We don't want to sound too gloomy here, and won't leave this topic without pointing you to places where you can find some of the triumphs of screening and case-finding: a good place to start is the Canadian Task Force on the Periodic Health Examination, where there are some rigorously evaluated ones.[4]

TIPS FOR TEACHING AROUND DIAGNOSTIC TESTS

We usually begin by asking learners why we perform diagnostic tests, because they often respond: "To find out what's wrong with the patient [dummy!]" This provides an opening for helping them to recognize that diagnosis is not about finding absolute truth but about limiting uncertainty, and establishes both the necessity and the logical base for introducing probabilities, pragmatic test–treatment thresholds, and the like. It's also a time to get them to start thinking about what they're going to do with the results of the diagnostic test and about whether doing the test will really help their patient (maybe they'll conclude that the test isn't necessary!).

When teaching about early diagnosis, we often challenge our learners with the statement: "Even when therapy is worthless, early diagnosis always improves survival!" and then help them recognize the distortions that arise from drawing conclusions about volunteers, from starting survival measurements unfairly early in screened patients, and from failing to recognize that early detection tests preferentially identify slowly – rather than rapidly – progressive disease. Once they've grasped those ideas, we think they're safe from the evangelists of early diagnosis.

References

1   Fleming K A. Evidence-based pathology. Evidence-Based Medicine 1997; 2: 132.

2   Richardson W S, Wilson M C, Guyatt G H, Cook D J, Nishikawa J, for the Evidence-Based Medicine Working Group. Users' guides to the medical literature: XV. How to use an article about disease probability for differential diagnosis. JAMA 1999; 281: 1214–9.

3   Macdonald L A, Sackett D L, Haynes R B, Taylor D W. Labelling in hypertension: a review of the behavioural and psychological consequences. J Chronic Dis 1984; 37(12): 933–42.

4   Canadian Task Force on the Periodic Health Examination. The periodic health examination. Can Med Assn J 1979; 121: 1193–254.

Further reading

Jaeschke R, Guyatt G H, Sackett D L for the Evidence-Based Medicine Working Group. Users' guides to the medical literature. VI. How to use an article about a diagnostic test: A: Are the results of the study valid? JAMA 1994; 271: 389–91.

Jaeschke R, Guyatt G H, Sackett D L for the Evidence-Based Medicine Working Group. Users' guides to the medical literature. VI. How to use an article about a diagnostic test: B. What are the results and will they help me in caring for my patients? JAMA 1994; 271: 703–7.

McGinn T, Randolph A, Richardson S, Sackett D. Clinical prediction guides. Evidence-Based Medicine 1998; 3: 5–6.

Sackett D L, Haynes R B, Guyatt G H, Tugwell P. Clinical epidemiology; a basic science for clinical medicine, 2nd edn. Little, Brown, Boston, 1991. *Chapter 4 on the interpretation of diagnostic data, and Chapter 5 on early diagnosis.*

Prognosis

As clinicians, we consider questions about prognosis all the time. Sometimes the questions are posed by patients and are quite direct: "How long have I got?". At other times, we pose these questions ourselves, and they may be less direct, as when deciding whether to treat at all (e.g. an elderly man with chronic lymphocytic leukemia who feels well – would his prognosis be importantly altered if he were left alone until he becomes symptomatic?) or deciding whether to screen (e.g. for abdominal aortic aneurysms – what is the fate of the undetected 4 cm aneurysm?). These questions share three elements: a qualitative aspect (Which outcomes could happen?), a quantitative aspect (How likely are they to happen?) and a temporal aspect (Over what time period?). In Chapter 1 we discussed how to recognize such questions about prognosis and in Chapter 2 we addressed how to find good information about prognosis. In this chapter, we'll present a framework for appraising the validity, importance and applicability of evidence about prognosis, using the same sorts of guides as we used in the chapter on diagnosis. When we're scanning articles about prognosis, we can use the first two validity guides for screening, selecting only those that pass both guides to spend more time on.

IS THIS EVIDENCE ABOUT PROGNOSIS VALID?

Table 4.1 Is this evidence about prognosis valid?

1. Was a defined, representative sample of patients assembled at a common (usually early) point in the course of their disease?

2. Was patient follow-up sufficiently long and complete?

3. Were objective outcome criteria applied in a 'blind' fashion?

4. If subgroups with different prognoses are identified:
   • Was there adjustment for important prognostic factors?
   • Was there validation in an independent group of 'test-set' patients?

1. Was a defined, representative sample of patients assembled at a common (usually early) point in the course of their disease?

Ideally, the prognosis study we find would include the entire population of patients who ever lived who developed the disease, studied from the instant of its onset. Because this ideal is impossible, we'll want to see how close the report we're reading approaches this ideal in terms of how the disease was defined and how the participants were assembled. If the study sample fully reflects the spectrum of illness we find in our own practice, we are reassured.

But when should the "clock" start? That is, from what point in the disease should patients be followed? If investigators begin tracking outcomes only *after* some patients have already finished their course with the disease, then the outcomes for these patients might never be counted. Some would have recovered quickly, while others might have died quickly. So, to avoid missing outcomes by "starting the clock" too late, we look to see that study patients were included at a uniformly early time in the disease, ideally when it first becomes clinically manifest; this is called an "inception cohort". An exception occurs when we want only to learn about the prognosis of a late stage in the disease; in this case we'd look for a representative and well-defined sample of patients who were all at a similarly advanced stage.

2. Was patient follow-up sufficiently long and complete?

Ideally, every patient in the inception cohort would be followed until they fully recover or develop one of the other disease outcomes. If a short follow-up led to just a few patients developing the outcomes of interest, we wouldn't have enough to go on when advising our patients. By the same token if, after years of follow-up, only a few adverse events have occurred, this good prognostic result is very useful in reassuring our patients about their future. But if the follow-up seems too short for the study patients to have developed a valid picture of the outcomes of interest, we'd better look for other evidence.

If the follow-up is long enough, we still have to worry about patients who entered the study but got lost along the way, as the reasons for their loss may be crucial. Some losses to follow-up are both unavoidable and mostly unrelated to prognosis (e.g. moving away to a different job or country) and these are not a cause for worry, especially if their numbers are small. But other losses might arise because patients die or are too ill to continue follow-up (or lose their independence and move in with family), and the failure to document and report their outcomes will reduce the validity of any conclusion the report draws about their prognosis.

Short of finding a report that kept track of every patient, how can we judge whether follow-up is "sufficiently complete"? There is no single answer for all studies, but we offer two suggestions to help. The first is a simple "5 and 20" rule: fewer than 5% loss probably leads to little bias, greater than 20% loss seriously threatens validity, and in-between amounts cause intermediate amounts of trouble. While this may be easy to remember, it may oversimplify for clinical situations in which the outcomes are infrequent. The second approach uses a simple sequence of "what if ... ?" questions, known as "sensitivity analysis".

Imagine a study of prognosis wherein 100 patients enter the study, four die and 16 are lost to follow-up. A "crude" case-fatality rate would count the four deaths among the 84 with full follow-up, or 4.8%. But what about the lost 16? Some or all of them might have died too. In a "worst case" scenario, all would have died, giving a case-fatality rate of (4 known + 16 lost) = 20 out of (84 followed + 16 lost), or 20/100, i.e. 20% – four times the rate reported in the study! Note that for the "worst case" scenario we've added the lost patients to both the numerator and the denominator of the outcome rate. On the other hand, in the "best case" scenario, none of the lost 16 would have died, yielding a case-fatality rate of 4 out of (84 followed + 16 lost), or 4/100, i.e. 4%. Note that for the "best case" scenario we've added the missing cases to just the denominator. While this "best case" of 4% may not differ much from the observed 4.8%, the "worst case" of 20% does differ meaningfully, and we'd probably judge that this study's follow-up was not sufficiently complete. By using this simple sensitivity analysis, we can see what effect losses to follow-up might have on study results, which can help us judge whether the follow-up was complete enough to yield valid results.

3. Were objective outcome criteria applied in a "blind" fashion?

Diseases affect patients in many important ways; some are easy to spot and some are more subtle. In general, outcomes at both extremes – death or full recovery – are relatively easy to detect with validity, but assigning a cause of death is often a matter of opinion (as anyone who has completed a death certificate knows!). In between these extremes are a wide range of outcomes that can be more difficult to detect or confirm, and where investigators will have to use judgment in deciding how to count them (e.g. readiness for return to work, or the intensity of residual pain). To minimize the effects of bias in measuring these outcomes, investigators should have established specific criteria that define each important outcome and then used them throughout patient follow-up. We'd want to satisfy ourselves that they are sufficiently objective for confirming the outcomes we're interested in. The occurrence of death is objective, but judging the underlying cause of death is very prone to error (especially when it's based on death certificates) and can be biased unless objective criteria are applied to carefully gathered clinical information.

But even with objective criteria, some bias might creep in if the investigators judging the outcomes also know about the patients' prior characteristics. In valid studies, investigators making judgments about clinical outcomes are kept "blind" to these patients' clinical characteristics and prognostic factors.

4. If subgroups with different prognoses are identified, was there adjustment for important prognostic factors and validation in an independent group of "test set" patients?

The final guide has to do with reports that claim that one subgroup of patients has a different prognosis from others. Such reports are common and for good clinical reason. Often we will want to know whether subgroups of patients have different prognoses (e.g. among patients with non-valvular atrial fibrillation, are those with enlarged left atria at higher risk of stroke than those with normal-sized atria?). First, we look to see whether there was adjustment for other important prognostic factors. That is, authors of these reports can make sure that these subgroup predictions are not being distorted by the unequal occurrence of another, powerful prognostic factor (such as would occur if patients with large atria were also more likely to have had prior embolic stroke than patients with normal atria). There are both simple (e.g. stratified analyses displaying the prognoses of patients with large atria separately for those with and without prior embolic stroke) and fancy (e.g. multiple regression analyses that can take into account not only prior embolic stroke but also hypertension, left ventricular function and the like) ways of adjusting for these other important prognostic factors. We can examine the methods and results sections to reassure ourselves that one or the other has been applied before we *tentatively* accept the conclusion about a different prognosis for the subgroup of interest.

We say "tentatively" because the statistics of determining subgroup prognoses are all about prediction, not explanation. They are indifferent to whether the prognostic factor is physiologically logical (in our running example, left atrial size) or a biologically nonsensical and random, non-causal quirk in the data (whether the patient lives on the north or the south side of the street). Putative prognostic factors can be demographic (such as age, gender, socioeconomic status), disease-specific (such as extent of disease, degree of test abnormality), or co-morbid (presence or absence of other conditions).

For this reason, the first time a prognostic factor is identified, there is no guarantee that it really does predict subgroups of patients with different prognoses. The initial patient group in which prognostic factors are found is called a "training set" or "derivation set". Because of the risk of spurious, chance nomination of prognostic factors, we should look to see whether the predictive power of such factors has been confirmed in subsequent, independent groups of patients, termed "test sets" or "validation sets". A good clue for this is a statement in the study's methods section of a pre-study intention to examine this specific group of prognostic factors, based on their appearance in a training set or previous study.

If a second, independent study validates the predictive power of prognostic factors, we have a very useful "clinical prediction guide" (CPG) of the sort that we met in Chapter 3, but this time predicting our patient's outcome after he or she is diagnosed.

If the evidence about prognosis appears valid after considering the above guides, we can turn to examining its importance and applicability. But if we find large potential for bias, we'd be better off searching for other evidence.

IS THIS VALID EVIDENCE ABOUT PROGNOSIS IMPORTANT?

Table 4.2 Is this valid evidence about prognosis important?

1. How likely are the outcomes over time?
2. How precise are the prognostic estimates?

1. How likely are the outcomes over time?

Once we're satisfied that an article's conclusions are valid, we can examine it further to see how likely each outcome is over time. Typically they are reported in three ways: as a percentage of survival at a particular point in time (such as 1-year or 5-year survival rates); as median survival (the length of follow-up by which 50% of study patients have died); or as survival curves that depict, at each point in time, the proportion (expressed as a percentage) of the original study sample who have NOT yet had a specified outcome. Figure 4.1 shows four survival curves, each leading to a different conclusion.

In panel A of Figure 4.1, virtually no patients have had events by the end of the study, so either prognosis is very good (in which case the study is very useful to us) or the study is too short (in which case it's not very useful). Panels B, C and D depict a serious disease, with only 20% of patients surviving at 1 year; we could tell such patients that their chances of surviving for a year are 20%. Note, however, that the shapes of these curves are quite different, so that the median survival (by which time half of them have succumbed) is 9 months for the disorder described in panel C but only 3 months for the

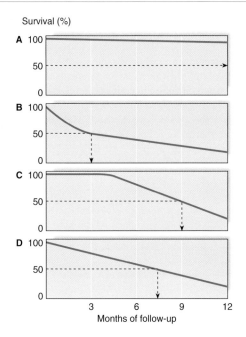

Figure 4.1 Prognosis shown as survival curves. **A:** Good prognosis (or too short a study!). **B:** Poor prognosis early, then slower increase in mortality, median survival of 3 months. **C:** Good prognosis early, then worsening, with median survival of 9 months. **D:** Steady prognosis.

disorder in panel B. The survival pattern is a steady, uniform decline only in panel D. Because 1-year survival, median survival and survival curves often tell us different things, a full picture of prognosis often requires all three.

2. How precise are the prognostic estimates?

As we pointed out earlier, investigators study prognosis in a sample of diseased patients, not the whole population of everyone who has ever had the disease. Purely by the play of chance, then, a study repeated 100 times among different batches of patients, even with identical entry characteristics, is bound to generate different estimates of prognosis. In deciding whether a given set of prognostic results is important, we need some means of judging just how much its results could vary by chance alone. By convention this is expressed as a 95% confidence interval, which represents the range of values within which we can be 95% sure that the population value lies. The narrower the confidence interval, the more assured we can feel about it. The text, tables or graphs of a proper prognostic study include the confidence intervals for its estimates of prognosis (and if they don't, you ought to be able to apply the appendix of this book and calculate the confidence interval for at least one of them yourself).

CAN WE APPLY THIS VALID, IMPORTANT EVIDENCE ABOUT PROGNOSIS TO OUR PATIENT?

Table 4.3 Can we apply this valid, important evidence about prognosis to our patient?

1. Are the study patients similar to our own?
2. Will this evidence make a clinically important impact on our conclusions about what to offer or tell our patient?

1. Are the study patients similar to our own?

This guide asks us to compare our patients with those in the article, using descriptions of the study sample's demographic and clinical characteristics. Inevitably, some differences will turn up, so how similar is similar enough? We recommend framing the question the other way: are the study patients so different from ours that we should not use the results at all in making predictions for our patients? As long as the answer to this question is "no", we can use the study results to inform our prognostic conclusions.

2. Will this evidence make a clinically important impact on our conclusions about what to offer or tell our patient?

If the evidence suggests an excellent prognosis when patients remain untreated, our discussions with patients would reflect these facts and would focus on whether any treatment should be started. If, on the other hand, the evidence suggests that the prognosis is gloomy without treatment (and if there are treatments that can make a meaningful difference), then our conversations with patients would reflect these facts and more likely lead us to treatment. Even when the prognostic evidence does not lead to a treat/don't treat decision, valid evidence can be useful in providing patients and families with the information they want about what the future is likely to hold for them and their illness.

Further reading

Christakis N A, Sachs G A. The role of prognosis in clinical decision making. J Gen Intern Med 1996; 11: 422–5.

Laupacis A, Wells G, Richardson W S, Tugwell P, for the Evidence-Based Medicine Working Group. Users' guides to the medical literature. V. How to use an article about prognosis. JAMA 1994; 272: 234–7.

Randolph A G, Guyatt G H, Richardson W S, for the Evidence-Based Critical Care Group. Prognosis in the intensive care unit: Finding accurate and useful estimates for counseling patients. Crit Care Med 1998; 26: 767–72.

Therapy

Having found some useful evidence about therapy, we have to decide where to start in the critical appraisal process. We could start by appraising its validity (arguing that if it isn't valid, who cares whether it appears to show a huge effect?). Alternatively, we could skip ahead and determine its clinical importance (arguing that if the evidence doesn't suggest a clinically important impact, who cares if it's valid?). We can start with either question, as long as we remember to follow up one favorable answer with the other question. To illustrate our discussion, we'll consider a patient with secondary progressive multiple sclerosis (MS) who is requesting interferon therapy, generating the clinical question: "In a patient with secondary progressive MS, will treatment with interferon decrease the risk of progression?" The CAT that we generated in answering this question appears on page 130, and you might want to refer to it along the way.

Types of therapeutic reports

This first section will help us assess evidence about therapy derived from individual reports. But we must always remember that they are not the best evidence we can find about the effects of therapy. When several randomized trials of the same treatment for the same condition have been carried out, an overview, which systematically reviews and combines all of them, would provide us with a better answer than the results from just one study. For this reason, we suggested in Chapter 2 that our literature searches should always begin with looking for systematic reviews, and the guides for determining their validity are in Table 5.9. However, because systematic reviews assess their component trials individually (and because we want to be sure that they've done so in a valid way), and since at this point in time we're more likely to find individual trials than systematic reviews, we'll begin with discussing the individual trial. Sometimes our literature search will yield a clinical decision analysis, and rules for deciding whether it's valid are presented in Table 5.15. Finally, we may track down an economic analysis, and questions that will help us decide whether we can believe the results are listed in Table 5.18.

REPORTS OF INDIVIDUAL STUDIES

Are the results of this individual study valid?

Table 5.1 Are the results of this individual study valid?

1. Was the assignment of patients to treatment randomized? And was the randomization list concealed?
2. Was follow-up of patients sufficiently long and complete?
3. Were all patients analyzed in the groups to which they were randomized?

Some less important points:

4. Were patients and clinicians kept blind to treatment?
5. Were groups treated equally, apart from the experimental therapy?
6. Were the groups similar at the start of the trial?

1. Was the assignment of patients to treatment randomized? And was the randomization list concealed?

When considering this, the most important question to ask is: Was the assignment of patients to treatment randomized? Did the investigators use some method analogous to tossing a coin* to assign patients to treatment groups (the experimental treatment is assigned if the coin landed "heads" and a conventional, "control" or "placebo"† treatment is given if the coin landed "tails")? The reason we should insist on random allocation to treatment is that this comes closer than any other research design to creating groups of patients at the start of the trial who are identical in their risk for the event we're hoping to prevent. Random allocation balances the groups for prognostic factors (such as disease severity or other

---

* In practice, the coin-tossing is done by computers but the principle remains the same.

† A placebo is a treatment that is so similar in appearance, taste etc. that the patient ("single-blind"), or the clinician, or both ("double-blind") are unable to distinguish it from the active treatment

predictors of especially good or bad prognosis) which, if they were unevenly distributed between treatment groups, could exaggerate, cancel or even counteract the effects of therapy.[‡] If these factors exaggerated the apparent effects of an otherwise ineffectual treatment, the effects of their imbalance could lead to the false-positive conclusion that the treatment was useful when in fact it wasn't. In contrast, if they cancelled or counteracted the effects of a really efficacious treatment, this could lead to false-negative conclusions that a useful treatment was useless or even harmful. Randomization balances the treatment groups for these factors, even if we don't yet know enough about the target disorder to know what they all are.

We should also look to see if randomization was concealed from the clinicians who entered patients into the trial. If it was concealed, the clinicians would be unaware of which treatment the next patient would receive and thus unable, consciously or unconsciously, to distort the balance between the groups being compared. As with failure to use random allocation, inadequate concealment of allocation can distort the apparent effect of treatment in either direction, causing the effect to seem larger or smaller than it really is.

Usually it is easy to tell whether a study was randomized because it is something to be proud of and the term might appear in its title or, most commonly, in its abstract. In contrast, it's not often stated whether the randomization list was concealed, but if randomization occurred by telephone or by some system that was at a distance from where patients were being entered into the trial, we can be assured by this. In the MS trial that we found to answer our question about the efficacy of interferon, the title states that it is a randomized trial and a quick scan of the methods tells us that randomization for this multicentre study was done at a central location.

[‡] A confounder is a name for these sorts of patient characteristics that are extraneous to the question posed, could cause the clinical events we are trying to prevent with the treatment, and might be unevenly distributed between the treatment groups. Although there are other easy ways of avoiding confounding (exclusion, stratified sampling, matching, stratified analysis, standardization and multivariate modeling), they all demand that we already know what the confounder is.

If the study wasn't randomized, we'd suggest that you stop reading it and go on to the next article in your search. Only if you can't find any randomized trials should you go back to it. If, however, the sole evidence you have about a treatment is from non-randomized studies, you have five options:

1. Check Chapter 2 again or get some help in doing another literature search to see if you missed any randomized trials of the therapy.

2. See whether the treatment effect is so huge that you can't imagine it could be a false-positive study (this option is very rare, and usually only satisfied when the prognosis of untreated patients is uniformly awful). As a check, you could ask several colleagues whether they consider the candidate therapy so likely to be efficacious that they'd consider it unethical to randomize a patient like yours into a study of it that includes a no-treatment or placebo group.

3. If the non-randomized trial concluded that the treatment was useless or harmful, then it is usually safe to accept that conclusion. This is because false-positive conclusions from non-randomized studies are far more common than false-negative ones (since treatments are typically withheld from patients with the poorest prognoses, and patients who faithfully take their medicine are destined for better outcomes, even when they are taking worthless treatments or placebos!).

4. Consider whether an "n-of-1" trial would make sense to you and your patient (Table 5.22).

5. Try to find evidence for some other treatment or simply provide supportive care.

2. Was follow-up of patients sufficiently long and complete?

Once we are satisfied that the study was randomized, we can look to see if all patients who were entered into the trial were accounted for at its conclusion. Ideally, we'd like to see that no patients have been lost to follow-up in the study because these patients could have had outcomes that would affect the conclusions of the study. If, for example, patients receiving the experimental treatment dropped out because of adverse outcomes, their absence from the analysis would lead to an overestimation of the efficacy of the treatment.

What can we consider to be an acceptable loss? To be sure of a trial's conclusion, the investigators should be able to take all patients who were lost to follow-up, assign them the worst case outcome (assume that everyone lost from the group whose remaining members fared better had a bad outcome and assume that everyone lost from the group whose remaining members fared worse had a rosy outcome), and still be able to support their original conclusion. It would be unusual for a trial to withstand a worst case analysis if it lost more than 20% of its patients and journals like *Evidence-Based Medicine* and *ACP Journal Club* won't publish trials with < 80% follow-up. Our interferon study had a > 90% follow-up.

We should also ensure that the follow-up of patients was sufficiently long to see a clinically important effect. For example, if our study assessing the use of interferon only followed patients up for 1 month, it's unlikely that we'd find the results helpful. Given the nature of the target disorder, we'd like to see a follow-up period of several months or, ideally, years. In our example, all patients had been in the interferon study for at least 2 years.

3. Were all patients analyzed in the groups to which they were randomized?

Because anything that happens after randomization can affect the chance that a study patient has an event, it's important that all patients (even those who fail to take their medicine or accidentally or intentionally receive the wrong treatment) are analyzed in the groups to which they were allocated. As we've already noted, it has been shown repeatedly that patients who "do" and "don't" take their study medicine have very different outcomes, even when the study medicine they have been prescribed is a placebo. To preserve the value of randomization, we should demand an "intention-to-treat analysis" whereby all patients are analyzed in the groups to which they were initially assigned, regardless of whether they received their assigned treatment. The interferon study did use an intention-to-treat analysis and we can feel confident that it has passed all three major validity criteria.

4. Were patients and clinicians kept blind to treatment?

5. Were groups treated equally, apart from the experimental therapy?

There are some less important points that we need to consider when appraising a study for validity. Were the patients and clinicians kept blind to the treatment? This is necessary to avoid the patient's reporting of symptoms or the clinician's interpretation of them being affected by hunches about whether the treatment is effective. The double-blind method also prevents patients and their clinicians from adding any additional treatments (or "co-interventions"), apart from the experimental treatment, to just one of the groups.

When patients and clinicians can't be kept blind (such as in surgical trials), often it is possible to have other, blinded clinicians assess clinical records (purged of any mention of treatment) or to make special, objective outcome measurements. Although the interferon study was a double-blind placebo-controlled trial, the fact that interferon injections often produce local reactions means that their physicians might have been able to guess which ones were receiving active treatment. We are reassured to learn that the outcomes in this study were determined by a different group of clinicians from those providing patient care.

6. Were the groups similar at the start of the trial?

Finally, we should check to see if the groups were similar in all prognostically important ways (except for receiving the treatment) at the start of the trial. And, if they weren't similar, was adjustment for these potentially important prognostic factors carried out? In the interferon study, there were no significant differences between patients receiving placebo and those receiving interferon.

Are the valid results of this individual study important?

In this section, we'll discuss how to determine if the potential benefits (or harms) of the treatment described in a study are important. We'll refer back to the guides in Table 5.2 for this

Table 5.2 Are the valid results of this individual trial important?

1. What is the magnitude of the treatment effect?
2. How precise is this estimate of the treatment effect?

discussion. Deciding whether we should be impressed with the results of a trial requires two steps: first, finding the most useful clinical expression of these results; and second, comparing these results with the results of other treatments for other target disorders.

1. What is the magnitude of the treatment effect?

There are a variety of methods that we can use to describe results, and we've included the most important ones in Table 5.3; once again, we'll illustrate them with the help of the interferon study. As you can see from the actual trial results in Table 5.3, by 33 months, progression of disability occurred among 50% of patients with multiple sclerosis randomized to the control group (we'll call this the "control event rate", CER) and in 39% of the patients assigned to receive interferon (we'll call this the "experimental event rate", EER). This difference was statistically significant, but how can it be expressed in a clinically useful way? Until recently, the usual measure of this effect reported in clinical journals was the relative risk reduction (RRR) calculated as (|CER − EER|/CER). In this example, the RRR is (50% − 39%)/50%, i.e. 22%, and we can say that interferon decreased the relative risk of progressing disability by 22%. In a similar way, we can describe the situation in which the experimental treatment increases the risk of a good event as the "relative benefit increase" (RBI; also calculated as |CER − EER|/CER). Finally, if the treatment increases the probability of a bad event we can use the same formulae to generate the "relative risk increase" (RRI).

One of the disadvantages of the RRR, which makes it unhelpful for our purposes, is revealed in the hypothetical bottom row of Table 5.3: it doesn't reflect the risk of the event without therapy (the CER, or baseline risk) and therefore cannot discriminate huge treatment effects from small ones. For example, if the rates of progression of disability were

Table 5.3 Clinically useful measures of the effects of treatment

	Event rate = progression of disability by 33 months		Relative risk reduction (RRR = ICER − EER/CER)	Absolute risk reduction (ARR = ICER − EERI)	Number needed to treat (NNT = 1/ARR)
	Control event rate (on placebo) (CER)	Experimental event rate (on interferon) (EER)			
In the actual trial Lancet 1998; 352: 1491−7	50%	39%	(50% − 39%)/50% = 22%	50% − 39% = 11%	1/11% = 9
In the hypothetical trivial case	0.00050%	0.00039%	(0.00050% − 0.00039%)/ 0.00050% = 22%I	0.00050% − 0.00039% = 0.00011%	1/0.00011% = 909 090

trivial (0.000 50%) in the control group and similarly trivial (0.000 39%) in the experimental group, the RRR remains 22%!

In contrast to this, the absolute risk reduction (the absolute arithmetic difference between the CER and EER) clearly does discriminate between these two situations and preserves the baseline risk. In the interferon trial, the ARR is 50% – 39% = 11%. In our hypothetical case where the baseline risk is trivial, the ARR is trivial, too, at 0.000 11%. Thus, the ARR is a more meaningful measure of treatment effects than is the RRR. When the experimental treatment increases the probability of a good event, we can generate the absolute benefit increase (ABI) which is also calculated by finding the absolute arithmetic difference in event rates. Similarly, when the experimental treatment increases the probability of a bad event, we can calculate the absolute risk increase (ARI).

However, ARRs may be difficult for us to remember (especially when they are less than 1.0). On the other hand, the inverse of the ARR (1/ARR) both is a whole number and has the useful property of telling us the number of patients that we need to treat (NNT) with the experimental therapy for the duration of the trial in order to prevent one additional bad outcome. In our example, the NNT is 1/11% = 9, which means we would need to treat nine people with interferon (rather than placebo) for 33 months to prevent one additional person from suffering a progression of their MS. In our hypothetical trivial example in the bottom row of Table 5.3, the clinical usefulness of the NNT is underscored, for this tiny treatment effect means that we would have to treat about a million (909 090) patients for 33 months to prevent one additional deterioration.

Should we be impressed with an NNT of 9? We can get an idea by comparing it with NNTs for other interventions and durations of therapy, tempered by our own clinical experience and expertise. We've provided some examples of NNTs in Table 5.4.[§] For example, we'd need to treat 29 people with

---

[§] A superb website that contains a host of relevant papers and hypertext links to a number of collections of NNTs has been developed by Andrew Booth at <http://www.shef.ac.uk/~scharr/ir/nnt.html>.

Table 5.4 Some useful NNTs[a]

Target disorder	Intervention	Events being prevented	Event rates		Follow-up time	Number needed to be treated (to prevent one event) (NNT)
			Control event rate (CER)	Experimental event rate (EER)		
Diabetes[b] (type 1)	Intensive insulin regimen	Diabetic neuropathy	9.6%	2.8%	6.5 years	15
Acute myocardial infarction[c]	Streptokinase infusion and daily aspirin thereafter	Death	13% 22%	8.1% 17%	5 weeks 2 years	19 24
Unstable angina[d]	Low-molecular-weight heparin (compared with unfractionated heparin)	Death, myocardial infarction (MI) or recurrent angina	23%	20%	30 days	29
Independent elderly people[e]	Comprehensive geriatric assessment	Long-term nursing home admission	10%	4%	3 years	17
Diastolic blood pressure 115–129 mmHg[f]	Antihypertensive drugs	Death, stroke, or MI	13%	1.4%	1.5 years	3
Diastolic blood pressure 90–109 mmHg[g]	Antihypertensive drugs	Death, stroke, or MI	5.5%	4.7%	5.5 years	128
Benign prostatic hypertrophy[h]	Finasteride	Surgery	10%	4.6%	4 years	18

Table 5.4 (cont'd)

| Target disorder | Intervention | Events being prevented | Event rates | | Follow-up time | Number needed to be treated (to prevent one event) (NNT) |
			Control event rate (CER)	Experimental event rate (EER)		
Healthy people with average total and LDL cholesterol and below-average HDL cholesterol[j]	Lovastatin	Fatal or non-fatal MI, or unstable angina, or sudden cardiac death	6%	4%	5.2 years	50
Non Q-wave myocardial infarction[j]	Conservative management	Death or non-fatal MI	22%	14%	1 year	13
Symptomatic high-grade carotid stenosis[k]	Endarterectomy (compared with best medical therapy)	Major stroke or death from any cause	18%	8%	2 years	10

[a]To find more examples, and to nominate additions to our databank of NNTs, refer to this textbook's website at: <http://www.library.utoronto.ca/medicine/ebm/>.

[b] Ann Intern Med 1995; 122: 561–8.
[d] JAMA 1997; 337: 447–52.
[f] JAMA 1967; 202: 116–22.
[h] NEJM 1998; 338: 557–63.
[j] NEJM 1998; 338: 1785–92.
[c] Lancet 1988; 2: 349–60.
[e] NEJM 1995; 333: 1184–9.
[g] BMJ 1995; 291: 97–104.
[i] JAMA 1998; 279: 1615–22.
[k] NEJM 1991; 325: 445–53

unstable angina with low-molecular-weight heparin to prevent one additional death or cardiac event at 30 days. In contrast, we'd have to treat over 100 people with hypertension for 5.5 years to prevent one death, stroke or MI. The NNT from our trial appears pretty impressive we think!

We can describe the adverse effects of therapy in an analogous fashion, as a number needed to harm one more patient (NNH) from the therapy. The NNH is calculated as 1/ARI. In the interferon study, only 37% of the control group experienced adverse events such as flu-like symptoms or necrosis at the injection site at some time during the 2-year study, whereas these events occurred in 64% of patients in the interferon group.** This absolute risk increase of |37% – 64%| = 27% generates an NNH over 33 months of 1/27% or 4. This means that we'd only need to treat four patients with interferon for 33 months to cause one additional patient to have an adverse event. Thus, the NNT and NNH provide us with a nice measure of the effort we and our patients have to expend to prevent or cause one more bad outcome, and their attractiveness as an effort:yield ratio (or "poor clinicians' cost-effectiveness analysis") is easily recognized. No wonder, then, that the NNT (and NNH) has come into such widespread use.

To understand NNTs, we need to consider two additional features. First, they always have a dimension of follow-up time associated with them. Quick reference to Table 5.4 reminds us that the NNT of 10 to prevent one more major stroke or death by performing endarterectomy on patients with symptomatic high-grade carotid stenosis refers to outcomes over a 2-year period (in this case, from an operation that is over in minutes). One consequence of this time dimension is that if we want to compare NNTs for different follow-up times we have to make an assumption about them and a "time adjustment" to at least one of them. Say that we wanted to compare the NNTs to prevent one additional stroke, MI or death with drugs among patients with mild versus severe

** We adopted a "worst case scenario" here by assuming that these adverse events occurred in different patients.

hypertension. Another quick look at Table 5.4 gives us an NNT at 1.5 years of just 3 for severe hypertensives (who already have a lot of target organ damage) and an NNT at 5.5 years of 128 for milder hypertensives (most of whom are free of target organ damage). To compare their NNTs we need to adjust at least one of them so that they relate to the same follow-up time. The assumption that we make here is that the RRR from treatment is constant over time (i.e. we assume that antihypertensive therapy exerts the same relative benefit in year 1 as it does over the next 4 years). If we are comfortable with that assumption (it appears safe for hypertension), we can then proceed to make the time adjustment. Let's adjust the NNT for the mild hypertensives (128 over the "observed" 5.5 years) to an NNT corresponding to a "hypothetical" 1.5 years. This is done by multiplying the NNT for the "observed" follow-up time by a fraction with the "observed" time in the numerator and the "hypothetical" time in the denominator. In this case, adjusting the NTT of 128 for mild hypertensives to its hypothetical value for 1.5 years becomes:

$$\text{NNT}_{\text{hypothetical}} = \text{NNT}_{\text{observed}} \times (\text{observed time/hypothetical time})$$

$$\text{NNT}_{1.5} = 128 \times (5.5/1.5) = 470$$

(By convention, we round any decimal NNT upwards to the next whole number.) Now we can appreciate the vast difference in the yield of clinical efforts to treat mild versus severe hypertensives: we need to treat 470 of the former, but only three of the latter for 1.5 years in order to prevent one additional bad outcome. The explanation lies in the huge difference in CERs (far higher in severe hypertensives followed just 1.5 years than in mild hypertensives followed 5.5 years), and nicely anticipates the modern guidelines for treating hypertension that take into account both target organ damage and the cardiovascular risk factors that raise CERs in deciding which subgroup of mild hypertensives to treat.

2. How precise is this estimate of the treatment effect?

The second thing we need to remember about the NNT is that, like any other clinical measure, NNTs are estimates of the truth and we should specify the limits within which we can confidently state the true NNT lies (if we want to specify the limits within which the true NNT lies 95% of the time, it's called specifying the 95% "confidence interval"). If you'd like to read more about confidence intervals, we refer you to Appendix 1. The smaller the number of patients in the study that generated the NNT, the wider its confidence interval, and even when the confidence interval is wide, it can provide us with some guidance.

The NNT is now in widespread use by journals and clinicians. However, the NNT and NNH fail to capture patients' individual likelihoods of benefit and harm. We'll discuss ways of capturing and incorporating these a bit later in this chapter (p. 123).

Are the valid, important results of this individual study applicable to our patient?

Now that we have decided that the evidence we have found is both valid and important, we need to consider if we can apply it to our own patient. The guides for doing this are in Table 5.5. To apply them, we need to integrate the evidence with our clinical experience and expertise, and with our patient's values and preferences.

1. Is our patient so different from those in the study that its results cannot apply?

Initially, we should consider whether our patient is so different from those in the study that its results don't apply. One approach would be to demand that our patient fit all the inclusion criteria for the study and to reject its usefulness if our patient didn't fit each and every one of them. This is not

Table 5.5 Are these valid, important results applicable to our patient?

1. Is our patient so different from those in the study that its results cannot apply?
2. Is the treatment feasible in our setting?
3. What are our patient's potential benefits and harms from the therapy?
4. What are our patient's values and expectations for both the outcome we are trying to prevent and the treatment we are offering?

a very sensible approach because most differences between our patients and those in trials tend to be quantitative (they have different ages or social classes or different degrees of risk of the outcome event or of responsiveness to the therapy) rather than qualitative (total absence of responsiveness or no risk of the event). We'd suggest that a far more appropriate approach is to consider whether our patient's sociodemographic features or pathobiology are so different from those in the study that its results are useless to us and our patient; only then should we discard its results and resume our search for relevant evidence. There are only a few occasions when this might be the case: different pharmacogenetics, absent immune responses, co-morbid conditions that prohibit the treatment, and the like. As a consequence of this clinical (as opposed to actuarial) approach, it's rare that we have to toss away a study for this reason. One difference we do need to consider is whether our patient is likely to accept our advice and comply with the demands of the therapeutic regimen, and we'll address that at the end of this section.

Sometimes treatments appear to produce qualitative differences in the responses of subgroups of patients so that they appear to benefit some subgroups but not others. Such qualitative differences in response are extremely rare. For example, even when some early trials of aspirin for transient ischemic attacks showed large benefits for men but none for women, subsequent trials and systematic reviews showed that this was a chance finding and that aspirin is efficacious in women. If you think that the treatment you're examining may work in a qualitatively different way among different subgroups of patients, you should refer to the guides in Table 5.6. To summarize them, unless the difference in response makes biological sense, was hypothesized before the trial, and has been confirmed in a second, independent trial, we'd suggest that you accept the treatment's overall efficacy as the best starting point for estimating its efficacy in your individual patient.

2. Is the treatment feasible in our setting?

Next we need to consider if the treatment is feasible in our practice setting. This includes determining whether our patient and our health care system can afford to pay for the treatment,

Table 5.6 Guides for whether to believe apparent qualitative differences in the efficacy of therapy in some subgroups of patients

A qualitative difference in treatment efficacy among subgroups is likely only when ALL the following questions can be answered "yes":

1. Does it really make biological and clinical sense?
2. Is the qualitative difference both clinically (beneficial for some but useless or harmful for others) and statistically significant?
3. Was it hypothesized before the study began (rather than the product of dredging the data) and has it been confirmed in other independent studies?
4. Was it one of just a few subgroup analyses carried out in the study?

its administration and monitoring, and any required follow-up. Interferon, for example, is currently "free" in some regions and countries but not in others, even on compassionate grounds.

3. What are our patient's potential benefits and harms from the therapy?

After we have decided that the study is applicable to our patients and that the treatment is feasible, we need to estimate our unique patient's benefits and risks of therapy. There are two general approaches to doing this. The first and longer approach begins by coming up with the best possible estimate of what would happen to our patient if he were not treated, his individual CER or "patient's expected event rate" (PEER). To this estimate we can then apply the overall RRR (for the events we hope to prevent with therapy) and RRI (for the side-effects of therapy) and generate the corresponding NNT and NNH for our specific patient. The second, much quicker approach skips this PEER step and works entirely from the study NNT and NNH. Both approaches assume that the relative benefits and risks of therapy are the same for patients with high and low PEERs. Because the second method is so much quicker, you might want to skip to page 121. If you want to learn the long way (first), read on.

The long way, via PEER. There are four ways to estimate our patient's PEER. First, we can simply assign our patient the overall CER from the study; that's easy, but sensible only if our patient is like the "average" study patient. Second, if the study has a subgroup of patients with characteristics similar to our own patient, we can assign the CER for that subgroup. (Indeed, in the unlikely event that we could say "yes" to all of the questions posed in Table 5.6, we could even apply the ARR for that subgroup to generate an NNT for our patient.) Third, if the study report includes a clinical prediction guide (validated in a second, independent study), we could use it to assign a PEER to our patient. Fourth, we could look for another paper that described the prognosis of untreated patients like ours (either in a simple form or in a multivariate prediction guide) and use its results to assign our patient a PEER.

All four methods we've described so far generate a PEER for our patient – what we would expect to happen to them if they received the "control" or comparison intervention in the study we're using. To convert this into an NNT or NNH for patients just like ours, we have to apply the corresponding RRR and RRI to them, using the formula:

$$NNT = 1/(PEER \times RRR)$$

For example, suppose that we find a paper that suggests that our MS patient has a risk of progression of disability of 80% (so the patient's PEER = 80%) over a period of time equal to the duration of the trial. The trial of interferon generated an overall RRR of 22%, so the NNT for patients like ours is $1/(80\% \times 22\%) = 6$. As you can see, these calculations can be cumbersome to do without a calculator, and fortunately Dr G Chatellier and his colleagues published the convenient nomogram shown in Figure 5.1 to help us.

The short way, sticking with NNT. The final method we can use to estimate an NNT for our patient is easier and faster, and this is the one we usually use at the bedside. In this approach, the estimate we make for our patient's risk of the outcome event (if the patient were to receive just the "control" therapy) is specified *relative to that of the average control patient*, and expressed as a "decimal fraction" we decided to call f_t. For example, if we think that our patient (if left untreated) has twice the risk of the outcome as control patients in the trial, $f_t = 2$; alternatively, if we think our patient is at only half

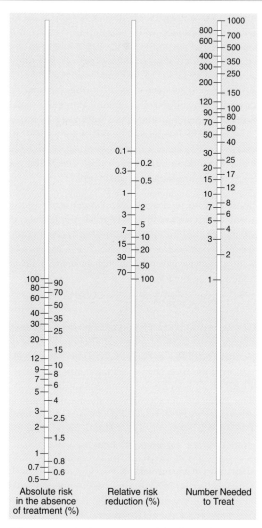

Figure 5.1 Nomogram for determining NNTs (Chatellier et al., BMJ 1996; 312: 426–9).

their risk, then $f_t = 0.5$. We can use past clinical experience and expertise in coming up with a value for f_t or we can use any of the information sources described in the previous section.

Remembering that all these methods assume the treatment produces a constant relative risk reduction across the range of susceptibilities, the NNT for patients just like ours is simply the reported NNT divided by f_t. In our interferon example, the study reported an NNT of 9, so that we'd need to treat nine MS patients like those in the trial with interferon for 33 months to prevent one more of them from progressing. If, however, we judge that our patient is at three times the risk of progressing without treatment as the patients in the control group of the study, $f_t = 3$ and $NNT/f_t = 9/3 = 3$. This means that we would only need to treat three higher-risk patients like ours for 33 months to prevent an additional one of them from progressing.

As before, we need to consider our patient's risk of adverse events from the therapy. To do this, we can use any of the same methods that we used to individualize our patient's NNT. Using the last and simplest one, where we generate an f_h, we may decide that our patient is at three times the risk of adverse events as patients in the control group of the study ($f_h = 3$), or we may decide that our patient is at one-third the risk ($f_h = 0.33$). Assuming the RRI of harm is constant over the spectrum of susceptibilities, we can adjust the overall study NNH of 4 with f_h (just as we did for the NNT), and generate NNH values of 1 and 12 corresponding to f_h values of 3 and 0.33, respectively.

4. What are our patient's values and expectations for both the outcome we are trying to prevent and the treatment we are offering?

Although the foregoing does a good job of individualizing the benefits and risks of therapy for our patient, it ignores his values and preferences. How can we incorporate these into a treatment recommendation? More importantly, how can we convert these into a form that permits our patient to make his own treatment decision? There are some beautifully elaborate ("Rolls Royce") ways of doing this, epitomized by formal clinical decision analysis (CDA), but they are prohibitively slow in the real world, as we'll describe in the section on CDA later in this chapter. Is there some quick way of accomplishing this (say, a "Ka" version) that doesn't do too much violence to the truth?

We'll show you the way that is used on the Sackett–Straus internal medicine in-patient service. It individualizes the patients' benefits and risks of therapy, incorporates their preferences, and informs them of the likelihood that the treatment will help vs. harm them. The key information required for this "likelihood of being helped vs. harmed" (LHH) is obtained in the course of informing patients about the bad outcomes we hope to prevent, and the adverse reactions we might cause, with therapy (something we should be doing anyway!). It goes like this:

Step 1: The first and critical step in this method is to elicit our patient's preferences. That is, we ask our patient to make value judgements about the relative severity of the bad outcome we hope to prevent with therapy and the adverse event we might cause with it. We begin this in the time-honored way of describing both of them, repeating these descriptions as needed after our patient has had the chance to think about them, and discuss them with family members, etc. When the treatment option is a common one (on our service, whether to take long-term warfarin for non-valvular atrial fibrillation), we might conclude our discussion by leaving our patient with a written description of the outcomes of foregoing and accepting the treatment. An example of what we would give a patient considering interferon for MS is shown in Table 5.7.

Following the review of these descriptions of the target event we hope to prevent and the side-effects we might cause, we work with the patient to help him express how severe he considers one of them relative to the other – is a relapse 20 times as severe as the side-effects? Five times as severe? This can be accomplished in a quick and simple way by asking our patient to tell us which is worse, and by how much. If the patient has difficulty making this comparison in a direct fashion, we present him with a rating scale (Fig. 5.2) the ends of which are anchored at 0 (= death[††]) and 1 (= full health). Next, we ask our patient to place a mark where he would consider the value of the target event we hope to prevent with

---

[††] Yes, our patients sometimes identify fates worse than death, in which case we extend the line below zero.

Table 5.7 Sample descriptions of the bad outcome we want to prevent and the potential adverse events we might cause with interferon

As we've discussed, multiple sclerosis is a disease that results in progressive disability. In your stage of disease, you may experience both relapses (sudden bursts when you have weakness or blurred vision, for example) and remissions of at least partial improvement. As the disease progresses, you will experience difficulty in doing things like walking, cooking, shopping and doing your banking. With further progression of the disease, you will have trouble talking, going to the toilet without someone helping you, and bathing and feeding yourself. Eventually you may need a wheelchair and a catheter in your bladder, and might have to be admitted to a chronic care facility.

There is a treatment called "beta-interferon" (which you could inject beneath your skin every other day) which may reduce your risk of these relapses and possibly this progression.

But this treatment has side-effects. You may develop flu-like symptoms at least once during your course of treatment. You also may develop a painful, reddened, swollen sore at the spot where you inject yourself.

treatment (our patient assigned disease progression a very low value of 0.05, almost as bad as being dead). Similarly, we ask him to place a second mark to correspond with his value for the adverse reactions to the treatment (our patient assigned the adverse events a value of 0.95, only a minor "disutility"). Comparing these two ratings, we can say that our patient believes that disease progression is 19 (0.95/0.05) times worse than the adverse events from the therapy. We then ask him whether this comparison makes sense, and usually repeat this process on a second occasion to see whether this relative severity is stable.

Step 2: To generate the LHH, we need to integrate our patient's values for these outcomes with the probability of their occurrence. As summarized in Table 5.8, we've

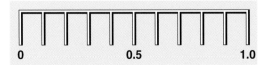

Figure 5.2 Rating scale for assessing values.

Table 5.8 Summary of risks and benefits of therapy

Outcome	Control event rate (CER)	Experimental event rate (EER)	Relative risk reduction (RRR)	Absolute risk reduction (ARR)	Number needed to treat (NNT)
Progression in disability	50% (or 1/2)	39% (or 1/2.5)	22%	11%	1/11% = 9
Outcome	CER	EER	Relative risk increase (RRI)	Absolute risk increase (ARI)	Number needed to harm (NNH)
Flu-like Illness or local reaction	37% (or 1/2.7)	64% (or 1/1.6)	73%	27%	1/27% = 4

already found that the average patient with MS has a 50% or a 1 in 2 chance of developing progression of the disease at 2 years, and that this can be decreased to 39% (roughly a 1 in 2.5 chance) with interferon (Table 5.8). The NNT for patients like those in the trial is 9 and if our patient is like them we can tell him that he has a 1 in 9 chance of being helped by interferon. Similarly, we noted that the average person in the control group had a 37% (or 1 in 2.7) chance of developing symptoms identical to those of a drug reaction during the trial, compared with 64% of people in the experimental group (or 1 in 1.6). The NNH for patients like those in the trial is 4, so that our patient can be told that he has a 1 in 4 chance of suffering an adverse event as a result of taking interferon.

This NNT and NNH can then be combined in an aggregate ratio, the likelihood of being helped versus harmed (LHH). To calculate this, we simply take the ratio of 1/NNT (remember this is the ARR) and 1/NNH (and this is the ARI). (For readers who prefer to work with ARRs and ARIs, we've repeated the following calculations in that format below.) For our patient, the first approximation of the LHH is:

$$LHH = (1/NNT) \text{ vs. } (1/NNH) = (1/9) \text{ vs. } (1/4) = 0.11 \text{ vs. } 0.25$$

i.e. 2:1 against interferon

As a first approximation, out patient can be told that "if you were like the patients in the trial, and if you felt that relapses and side-effects were of the same severity, interferon treatment is twice as likely to harm you as to help you".

But of course, this first approximation not only ignores our patient's unique individual risks for this benefit and harm (i.e. his PEERs for these events) but also omits our patient's preferences (or "utilities") for the outcome we are trying to prevent vs. the adverse events we may cause with therapy. We can most quickly particularize the former by employing the "f" method we described previously. Suppose, for example, that we judge our patient to be at three times the risk of a progression in disability ($f_t = 3$) but at about the same risk as those in the trial of an adverse event ($f_h = 1$). The risk-adjusted LHH becomes:

$$LHH = [(1/NNT) \times f_t] \text{ vs. } [(1/NNH) \times f_h]$$
$$= [(1/9) \times 3] \text{ vs. } [(1/4) \times 1]$$
$$= 1/3 \text{ vs. } 1/4, \text{ i.e. } 1.3:1$$

If that were the end of it, we could now tell our patient that "interferon is as likely to help you as to harm you" (note that we multiply, rather than divide, by f in this case because we are adjusting 1/NNT).

This risk-adjusted LHH still ignores our patient's values, so we further refine it by incorporating these. Remembering that our patient said that disease progression was at least 19 times worse than the adverse effects of interferon, we can designate this relative difference the "severity" factor (s) and use it to make our final adjustment in the LHH:‡‡

$$[(1/NNT) \times f_t \times s] \text{ vs. } [(1/NNH) \times f_h]$$
$$= [(1/9) \times 3 \times 19] \text{ vs. } [(1/4) \times 1]$$
$$= 6.3 \text{ vs. } 0.25, \text{ i.e. } 25:1$$

Thus, in the final analysis our patient is 25 times as likely to be helped vs. harmed by interferon. This LHH can then be presented to the patient, and he can decide whether it is favorable enough to offset the pain and hassle of having to inject himself with interferon every other day.

This example, in which the crude LHH of 2:1 against interferon was progressively refined to 1:1 and ultimately 25:1 in favor of interferon highlights how important it is to incorporate patients' unique risks and preferences into decisions about their care. If, for example, our patient was extremely risk-averse and thought that the adverse events were 10 times worse than the relapse we were hoping to prevent, the LHH would be $[(1/9) \times 3]$ vs. $[(1/4) \times 1 \times 10] = 0.33$ vs. 2.5, i.e. 1:8, and such a patient would be eight times as likely to be harmed vs. helped by interferon.

Repeating the foregoing discussion in the ARR format, the crude LHH = ARR vs. ARI = 11% vs. 27%, i.e. 2:1 against

---

‡‡ Note that the "s" factor is placed on the side of the LHH with the less desirable outcome (if the patient judges the side-effect to be worse than the event prevented by treatment, the "s" goes on the NNH side of the equation).

interferon. Incorporating our judgements that our patient is three times as likely to progress but equally likely to have an adverse reaction, the partially adjusted LHH = 11% × 3 vs. 27% = 33% vs. 27%, i.e. 1.3:1. Finally, incorporating our patient's preference (that progression was 19 times as bad as an adverse reaction), the fully adjusted LHH = (11% × 3 × 19) vs. 27% = 627% vs. 27%, i.e. 25:1, and interferon is 25 times as likely to help vs. harm our patient.

If we are unsure of our patient's "f" for benefit or harm, or if our patient is uncertain about his "severity" factor, we can come back later or do a sensitivity analysis. That is, we could insert other clinically sensible values for "f" and "s" and see how they affect the size and direction of the LHH.

The foregoing discussion demonstrates the "Ka" model of the LHH, but it is a far cry from the "Rolls Royce" of clinical decision analysis (a later section of this chapter deals with "CDA" – p. 138). We could add a few features to the basic LHH, making it into a Jaguar that can compare two active treatments (instead of just a placebo vs. experimental treatment as in our example). And, if there were several serious adverse events that could result from the treatment(s), we could add each of them to generate the fully adjusted LHH. Finally, as we will describe later in this chapter, we can also discount future events as in a CDA.

We've found that the LHH can be used in the busy clinical setting (median time to complete of 6.5 minutes), is intelligible to both clinicians and patients, and is unambiguously patient-centered. As other approaches in this rapidly developing field are validated in clinical settings they will appear on our website and in future editions of this book.

Now have a look at the CAT we generated on whether treatment with interferon will decrease the risk of progression of secondary progressive MS.

A WORD ON QUALITATIVE LITERATURE

In this book, we've focused primarily on searching for and appraising quantitative literature. Qualitative research may

CAT Multiple sclerosis – interferon delays progression

> **Clinical bottom line** Multiple sclerosis – interferon β-1b reduced the progression of secondary progressive MS.

Citation(s). European study group on interferon β-1b in secondary progressive MS. Placebo-controlled multicentre randomized trial of interferon β-1b in treatment of secondary progressive multiple sclerosis. Lancet 1998; 352: 1491–7.

Three-part clinical question. In patients with secondary progressive multiple sclerosis (MS), does interferon delay the progression of disability?

Search terms: "interferon" and "multiple sclerosis" in MEDLINE (but will be in Best Evidence 4).

The study
Double-blinded concealed randomized controlled trial with intention-to-treat analysis.

The study patients. Clinically or laboratory confirmed MS with secondary progression (a period of deterioration, independent of relapses, sustained for at least 6 months, following a period of relapsing-remitting MS), aged 18–55 years, with baseline Kurtzke Expanded Disability Scores (EDSS) of 3–6.5 and a history of at least two relapses or an increase of at least 1 point on the EDSS in the previous 2 years. Patients were excluded if they had recently used immunosuppressive or immunomodulatory treatment or other putative agents. Steroids could be used for relapses.

Control group (n = 358; 358 analyzed). Standard care and placebo injection SQ

Experimental group (n = 360; 360 analyzed). 4 million IU interferon SQ on alternate days for 2 weeks and then 8 million IU on alternate days

The evidence

Outcome	Time to outcome	CER	EER	RRR	ARR	NNT
Progression of disability	33 months	0.498	0.389	22%	0.109	9
95% confidence intervals				7–36%	0.037–0.181	6–27
Patients wheelchair-bound	33 months	0.246	0.167	32%	0.079	13
95% confidence intervals				8–56%	0.020–0.138	7–50

Comments
1. Assessment of EDSS was done by different physicians from those who provided general patient care.
2. Physicians were trained in using the EDSS at a central reference center.
3. Interferon did cause adverse effects such as local reaction at injection site with an NNH of 4.
4. More patients in the placebo group received steroids.
5. This is the first study to show the effectiveness of interferon therapy in secondary-progressive MS and there are currently other studies underway that will hopefully confirm this finding, so this CAT needs to be reviewed/updated every 6 months.

Appraised by: SE Straus.   *Kill or update by:* 2000.

provide us with some guidance in deciding whether we can apply the findings from qualitative studies to our patients. The purpose of qualitative research is to understand phenomena in natural rather than experimental settings with emphasis on understanding the experiences and values of our patients. For example, returning to our patient with MS, we might want to look for studies that describe the experiences and feelings of patients with MS who have taken interferon or we might want to explore literature describing why patients might not comply with interferon therapy. The field of qualitative research has an extensive history in the social sciences but its exploration and development are relatively new to clinical medicine. We don't consider ourselves experts in this area and suggest that you take a look at the references we've included at the end of this section.

Further reading about individual randomized trials

Dans A L, Sand L F, Guyatt G H, Richardson W S for the Evidence-Based Medicine Working Group. Users' guides to the medical literature. XIV. How to decide on the applicability of clinical trial results to your patient. JAMA 1998; 279: 545–9.

Guyatt G H, Sackett D L, Cook D J for the Evidence-Based Medicine Working Group. Users' guides to the medical literature. II. How to use an article about therapy or prevention. A. Are the results of the study valid? JAMA 1993; 270: 2598–601.

Guyatt G H, Sackett D L, Cook D J for the Evidence-Based Medicine Working Group. Users' guides to the medical literature. II. How to use an article about therapy or prevention. B. What were the results and will they help me in caring for my patients? JAMA 1994; 271: 59–62.

Sackett D L, Haynes R B, Guyatt G H, Tugwell P. Clinical epidemiology. A basic science for clinical medicine, 2nd edn. Little, Brown, Boston, 1991.

Straus S E, Moore R A, McQuay H, Sackett D L. A proposed patient-centered method for describing the risks of benefit and harm from therapy: the likelihood of being helped versus harmed. In press.

Further reading about qualitative studies

Mays N, Pope C (eds). Qualitative research in health care. BMJ Publishing, London, 1996.

COMPLIANCE

Given that our patient accepts a favorable LHH and embarks on treatment, everything we and the patient have invested in diagnosis, critical appraisal, and individualizing the benefits and risks of therapy comes to naught if the patient can't or won't follow his regimen of medication taking, diet, exercise, and the like. We call this patient behavior "compliance", and stress that our use of the term carries no implications imperialistic clinicians or submissive patients. There is plenty written about compliance, and we'll summarize it only briefly here.

Compliance is a major problem in clinical and other types of health care. The usual compliance is about 50% for both short- and long-term treatments (with a range of 0–100+++% and considerable variation within patients from week to week). The causes for non-compliance are often not the ones we might think: age, sex, race, intelligence and education are not important. On the other hand, long waiting times, high cost, long duration and high complexity of treatments all lead to low compliance.

We should look for low compliance any time a patient fails to reach a treatment goal (and especially before we increase a dose or add another drug). Irregular appointment keeping is a major clue, and a positive response to a single question, "Have you missed one or more doses of your medication?", when asked in a non-threatening way, generates a LR+ of 4.4 for low compliance (and a LR– of 0.5). If uncertainty persists we can employ more expensive methods such as counting pills, checking pharmacy records (for refills), measuring drug levels in body fluids, and even providing special pill containers that keep a time record of dosing.

Our objective in detecting low compliance is to offer our patients strategies that might help them to comply.[§§] Several compliance-improving strategies have been validated in randomized trials, but none leads to huge improvements. For short-term treatments they comprise exact instructions, preferably backed up by written information. For long-term care they include complex combinations of greater attention

---

[§§] Before doing so, we ought to rethink the regimen and convince ourselves that it really is worth following.

and supervision: more convenient care, information on the exact regimen (but not a detailed explanation of the disease, unless the patient wants one), counseling, reminders, self-monitoring, reinforcement, and family therapy. The best summaries of compliance-improving strategies appear in the Cochrane Library, and were being updated as this book went to press.

Further reading about compliance

Haynes R B, McKibbon K A, Kanani R, Brouwers M C, Oliver T. Interventions to assist patients to follow prescriptions for medications. (Cochrane Review). The Cochrane Library (issue 2). Update Software, Oxford, 1999.

Stephenson B J, Rowe B H, Macharia W M, Leon G, Haynes R B. Is this patient taking their medication? JAMA 1993; 269: 2779–81.

REPORTS OF SYSTEMATIC REVIEWS

In one sense, this section is out of order, for the first target of any search about therapy should be a systematic review. This is because the systematic review of the effects of health care is the most powerful and useful evidence available. However, because the critical appraisal of a systematic review requires the skill to appraise the individual trials that comprise it, we've switched the order in this book.

A systematic review (SR) is a summary of the medical literature that uses explicit methods to systematically search, critically appraise, and synthesize the world literature on a specific issue. Its goal is to minimize both bias (usually by not only restricting itself to randomized trials, but also seeking published and unpublished reports in every language) and random error (by amassing very large numbers of individuals). SRs may, but need not, include some statistical method for combining the results of individual studies (and we'll call this subset "meta-analyses"). The guides that we consider when appraising a SR follow. Not surprisingly, many of them (especially around importance and applicability) are the same as those for individual reports, but those for validity are different.

Are the results of this systematic review valid?

Table 5.9 Guides for deciding whether the results of this systematic review are valid

1. Is this a systematic review of randomized trials?
2. Does this systematic review have a "methods" section that describes:
   - finding and including all relevant trials
   - how the validity of the individual studies was assessed?
3. Were the results consistent from study to study?

A less frequent point:

4. Were individual patient data used in the analysis (or aggregate data)?

Initially we need to determine whether the systematic review combines randomized or non-randomized trials. We've mentioned previously in this chapter the ability of the randomized trial to reduce bias. SRs, by combining all relevant randomized trials, further reduce both bias and random error and thus provide the highest level of evidence currently achievable about the effects of health care.*** In contrast, systematic reviews of non-randomized trials can compound the problems of individually misleading trials and produce a lower quality of evidence. For this reason, if the SR we find includes both randomized and non-randomized trials, we avoid it unless it separates these types of trials in its analyses.

We need to scrutinize the SR's methods section to determine whether it describes how the investigators found all the relevant trials. If not, we drop it at once and continue looking. If they did carry out a search, we seek reassurance that it went beyond standard bibliographic databases, as these have been shown to fail correctly to label up to half of the published trials in their own files. A more rigorous SR would include hand-searching journals (the starting point for any Cochrane Review), conference proceedings, theses, and the databanks of pharmaceutical firms, and contacting authors of published articles. Negative trials are less likely to be submitted and

---

*** That's why the Cochrane Collaboration has been likened in importance to the Human Genome Project.

selected for publication (which could result in a false-positive conclusion in a SR restricted to published trials) and the other sources regularly turn up less enthusiastic unpublished trials. Moreover, if the SR's authors restricted their search to reports in just one language, we need to recognize that this, too, could bias the conclusions. It has been observed, for example, that bilingual German investigators were more likely to submit trials with positive results to English language journals and those with negative results to German language journals. [†††]

The "methods" section of the report should also include a statement describing how the investigators assessed the validity of the individual studies (using criteria like those in Table 5.1). We would feel most confident in the systematic review in which multiple independent reviews of individual studies were carried out and showed good agreement.

Satisfied with the methods, we then need to address the SR's results. Were the effects of treatment consistent from study to study? We're more likely to believe the results of a systematic review if the results of every trial in it show a treatment effect that is at least going in the same direction (what we'd call "qualitatively" similar results). We shouldn't expect them to show exactly the same degree of efficacy (or "quantitatively identical" result), but we should be concerned if some trials confidently conclude a beneficial effect of treatment and others in the same review powerfully exclude any benefit or demonstrate a clear-cut harm. Moreover, we'd like to find that the investigators tested their results to see whether any lack of consistency (or "heterogeneity") was unlikely to be due to the play of chance. And, if they did find statistically significant heterogeneity, did they satisfactorily explain why it was observed (as differences in study patients, in doses of medications, in durations of therapy, and the like)?

A less frequent point to consider is whether the authors used individual patient data (rather than summary tables or published reports) for their analysis. We'd feel more confident about the conclusions of the study, especially as it related to

---

[†††] This observation applies to allopathic remedies; the situation is reversed for trials involving alternative medical therapies!

subgroups, if individual patient data were used, because they provide the opportunity to test promising subgroups from one trial in an identical subgroup from other trials (you might want to refer back to Table 5.6). Individual patient data also allow more reliable analyses of patients' time to specific clinical events.

Are the valid results of this systematic review important?

Table 5.10 Guides for deciding whether the valid results of this systematic review are important

1. What is the magnitude of the treatment effect?
2. How precise is the treatment effect?

Just as we examined the results of single therapeutic trials, we need to find a clinically useful expression for the results of systematic reviews, and here we become victims of history and some high-level statistics (the toughest in this book). Although growing numbers of SRs present their results as NNTs, most of them still use odds ratios (ORs) or relative risks (RRs).‡‡‡ Earlier in this chapter, we showed that the RRR doesn't preserve the control event rate (CER) or the patient's expected event rate (PEER), and this disadvantage extends to odds ratios and relative risks. Fortunately, although ORs and RRs are of very limited use in the clinical setting, they can be converted to NNTs (or NNHs) using the formulae in Table 5.11. Better

Table 5.11 Formulae to convert odds ratios (ORs) and relative risks (RRs) to NNTs

For RR < 1:
NNT = 1/(1 − RR) × PEER

For RR > 1:
NNT = 1/(RR − 1) × PEER

For OR < 1:
NNT = 1 − [PEER × (1 − OR)]/(1 − PEER) × (PEER) × (1 − OR)

For OR > 1:
NNT = 1 + [PEER × (OR − 1)]/(1 − PEER) × (PEER) × (OR − 1)

‡‡‡ An odds ratio is the odds of an event in a patient in the experimental group relative to that of a patient in the control group. Relative risk is the risk of an event in a patient in the experimental group relative to that of a patient in the control group.

yet, we've provided the results of some typical conversions in Tables 5.12 and 5.13.

Table 5.12 Translating odds ratios (ORs) to NNTs when OR <1[a]

		Odds ratio (OR) <1				
		0.9	0.8	0.7	0.6	0.5
Patient's	0.05	209[b]	104	69	52	41[c]
expected	0.10	110	54	36	27	21
event	0.20	61	30	20	14	11
rate	0.30	46	22	14	10	8
(PEER)	0.40	40	19	12	9	7
	0.50	38	18	11	8	6
	0.70	44	20	13	9	6
	0.90	101[d]	46	27	18	12[e]

[a] The numbers in the body of the table are the NNTs for the corresponding ORs at that particular PEER. This table applies when a bad outcome is prevented by therapy.
[b] The relative risk reduction (RRR) here is 10%.
[c] The RRR here is 49%.
[d] The RRR here is 1%.
[e] The RRR here is 9%.

Table 5.13 Translating odds ratios to NNTs or NNHs when OR >1

		Odds ratio (OR) >1				
		1.1	1.2	1.3	1.4	1.5
Patient's	0.05	212	106	71	54	43
expected	0.10	112	57	38	29	23
event	0.20	64	33	22	17	14
rate	0.30	49	25	17	13	11
(PEER)	0.40	43	23	16	12	10
	0.50	42	22	15	12	10
	0.70	51	27	19	15	13
	0.90	121	66	47	38	32

The numbers in the body of the table are the NNTs for the corresponding ORs at that particular PEER. This table applies both when a good outcome is increased by therapy and when a side-effect is caused by therapy. (Adapted from John Geddes, personal communication, 1999.)

We interpret the NNTs and NNHs derived from SRs in the same as we would for individual trials.

Are the valid, important results of this systematic review applicable to our patient?

Table 5.14 Guides for deciding whether the valid, important results of this systematic review are applicable to our patient

1. Is our patient so different from those in the study that its results cannot apply?
2. Is the treatment feasible in our setting?
3. What are our patient's potential benefits and harms from the therapy?
4. What are our patient's values and preferences for both the outcome we are trying to prevent and the side-effects we may cause?

A SR provides an overall, average effect of therapy which may be derived from a quite heterogeneous population. How do we apply this evidence to our individual patient? The same way we did it for individual trials – by applying the guides for applicability listed in Table 5.5. One advantage that SRs have over most randomized trials is that the former may provide precise information on subgroups which will help us to individualize the evidence to our own patients. In order to do this, however, we need to remind ourselves of the cautions about subgroups we've summarized in Table 5.6.

Further reading about systematic reviews

Chalmers I, Altman D (eds). Systematic reviews. BMJ Publishing, London, 1995.

Mulrow C, Cook D (eds) Systematic reviews. American College of Physicians, Philadelphia, 1998.

Oxman A D, Cook D J, Guyatt G H for the Evidence-Based Medicine Working Group. Users' guides to the medical literature. VI. How to use an overview. JAMA 1994; 272: 1367–71.

REPORTS OF CLINICAL DECISION ANALYSES

Occasionally, when we are attempting to answer a question about therapy, the results of our search will yield a clinical decision analysis (CDA). A CDA applies explicit, quantitative methods to compare the likely consequences of pursuing different treatment strategies. A CDA starts with a diagram called a "decision tree" which illustrates the target disorder, the alternative treatment strategies and their possible outcomes. A simple example is shown in Figure 5.3, which looks at the possible strategies for the management of atrial fibrillation, including anticoagulation, antiplatelet therapy, no antithrombotic prophylaxis, and electrical cardioversion. The point at which a treatment decision is made is marked

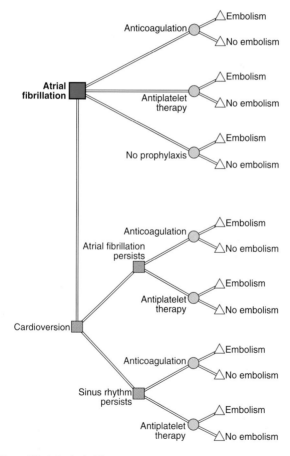

Figure 5.3 A simple decision tree.

with a box. The possible outcomes that arise from the treatment strategies follow this decision node and are preceded by circles, called "chance nodes". The probabilities for each of these events are estimated from the literature (hopefully with a modicum of accuracy!) or occasionally from the clinician's clinical expertise. Triangles are placed at the end of each outcome branch and the patient's utility for each outcome is placed here. A utility is the measure of a person's preference for a health state and is usually expressed as a decimal from 0 to 1. Typically, perfect health is assigned a value of 1 and death is assigned a value of 0, although there are some outcomes that patients may think are worse than death and the scale may need to be extended below zero. Sometimes CDAs may use life-years, quality-adjusted life-years (QALYs, where a year in a higher-quality health state contributes more to the outcome than a year in a poor-quality health state), or cases of disease or complications that are prevented. The utility of each outcome is multiplied by the probability that it will occur and this is summed for each chance node in the treatment branch to generate an average utility for that branch of the tree. The "winning" strategy, and preferred course of clinical action, is the one that leads to the highest utility.

On the authors' clinical services we've encountered an insurmountable time barrier to their use. To be done right, they have to generate and integrate probabilities and patient utilities for all the pertinent outcomes, and particularize these probabilities and utilities to a specific patient. The result is elegant, and we sometimes wish we could do it for all our patients, but the process takes us an average of 3 days to complete for just one of them.[§§§] A simple calculation for the last month on the Sackett–Straus service when we admitted 220 patients shows that we generated $220 \times 3 = 660$ days of CDAs to perform, but only 30 days in which to perform them. The alternatives were to hire 22 full-time decision analysts or to employ the more rough-and-ready but humanly feasible approaches for integrating evidence and patients' values such as the LHH we described in the section on individual

---

[§§§] And some clinical friends who are much more expert in CDA tell us we are faster than they are!

randomized trials. We chose the latter, and don't consider ourselves experts at CDA; if you are interested in reading more about how to do them, check out the references at the end of this section.

But even if we don't do CDAs, we sometimes read reports of them, and the rest of this section will describe how we decide whether they are valid, important, and applicable to a patient. The guides that we use to do this follow.

Are the results of this CDA valid?

Table 5.15 Guides for deciding whether the results of this CDA are valid

1. Were all important therapeutic alternatives (including no treatment) and outcomes included?
2. Are the probabilities of the outcomes valid and credible?
3. Are the utilities of the outcomes valid and credible?
4. Was the robustness of the conclusion tested?

The CDA should include all the treatment strategies and the full range of outcomes (both good and bad) that we think are important. For example, if we are interested in looking at a CDA that might help us determine the best management of non-valvular atrial fibrillation and the CDA we find doesn't include aspirin as an alternative treatment to anticoagulants, we should be skeptical about its usefulness (since both work, albeit to different degrees).

A CDA that is well done should explicitly describe a sensible, systematic process that was used to identify, select and combine the best external evidence into probabilities for all the important clinical outcomes. It should document a systematic literature search (see Ch. 2 for details) for all relevant evidence. There may be some uncertainty around a probability estimate and the authors should specify a range; this may come from the range of values from different studies or from a 95% confidence interval from a single study or systematic review. The methods that were used to assess the evidence for validity (see p. 106) should also be included in the study. If a systematic review was not found to provide an estimate of the probability, were the results of the studies that were found combined in some sensible way? For example, did the investigators perform a meta-analysis or a weighted average based on sample size or study quality? Finally, some investigators may use expert opinion to generate probability estimates, if these aren't available in the clinical literature, and these estimates won't be as valid as those obtained from evidence-based sources.

Were the utilities obtained in an explicit and sensible way from valid sources? Ideally, utilities are measured in patients using valid, standardized methods such as the standard gamble or time trade-off techniques. Occasionally, investigators will use values already present in the clinical literature or values obtained by "consensus opinion" from experts. These latter two methods are not nearly as credible as measuring utilities directly in patients.

Ideally, in a high-quality CDA, the investigators should "discount" future events. For example, most people wouldn't trade a year of perfect health now for one 20 years in the future – we usually value the present greater than the future. Discounting the utility will take this into account.

Finally, we need to look to see whether the CDA includes a sensitivity analysis. Were clinically sensible ranges of probabilities and utilities inserted into the CDA to see if the conclusion changed? This is done to test the robustness of the CDA.

If we think the CDA has satisfied all of the above criteria, we move on to considering whether the results of this CDA are important. If it doesn't satisfy the criteria, we'll have to go back to our search.

Are the valid results of this CDA important?

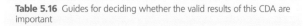

Table 5.16 Guides for deciding whether the valid results of this CDA are important

1. Did one course of action lead to clinically important gains?
2. Was the same course of action preferred despite clinically sensible changes in probabilities and utilities?

Was there a clear "winner" in this CDA, so that one course
of action clearly led to a higher average utility? Surprisingly,
experts in this area often conclude that average gains in
QALYs of as little as 2 months are worth pursuing (especially
when their confidence intervals are big, so that some patients
enjoy really big gains in QALYs). On the other hand, gains of
a few days to a few weeks are usually considered "toss-ups" in
which both courses of action lead to identical outcomes and
there is nothing to choose between them.

Before accepting the results of a positive CDA we need to
make sure it determined whether clinically sensible changes
in probabilities or utilities altered its conclusion. If this
"sensitivity analysis" generated no switch in the designation of
the preferred treatment, it is a robust analysis. If, on the other
hand, the designation of the preferred treatment is sensitive
to small changes in one or more probabilities or utilities, the
results of the CDA are uncertain and it may not provide any
important guidance for our patient and us.

Are the valid, important results of this CDA applicable to our patient?

Table 5.17 Guides for deciding whether the valid, important results of
this CDA are applicable to our patient

1. Do the probabilities in this CDA apply to our patient?
2. Can our patient state his/her utilities in a stable, useable form?

Once we've decided that the conclusions of a CDA are
both valid and important, we still need to decide whether
we can apply it to our patient. Are our patient's probabilities
of the various outcomes included in the sensitivity analysis?
If they lie outside the range tested, we'll need to either
recalculate it or at least be very cautious in following its
recommendations.

Similarly, we might want to generate utilities for our patient to
see if they fall within the range tested in the CDA. A crude
technique that we use on our clinical service begins by
drawing a line on a sheet of paper with two anchor points on

it: one at the top labeled "perfect health" which is given a value of 1, and one near the bottom labeled "death" which is given a score of 0 (making it precisely 10 or 20 cm long helps, as you'll see). After explaining it, we ask the patient to make a mark at the places on the scale that correspond to his current state of health and to all the other outcomes that might result from the choice of interventions. The locations that the patient selects are used to represent the utilities (if time permits, we leave the scale with the patient so that he can reflect on, and perhaps revise, the utilities). We can then see whether our patient's utilities (both initially and on reflection) lie within the boundaries of the study's sensitivity analysis.

Further reading about clinical decision analysis

Friedland D J, Go A S, Davoren J B, Shlipak M G, Bent S W, Subak L L, Mendelson T. Evidence-based medicine. A framework for clinical practice. Appleton & Lange, Stamford, 1998.

Richardson W S, Detsky A S for the Evidence-Based Medicine Working Group. Users' guides to the medical literature. VII. How to use a clinical decision analysis. A. Are the results of the study valid? JAMA 1995; 273: 1292–5.

Richardson W S, Detsky A S for the Evidence-Based Medicine Working Group. Users' guides to the medical literature. VII. How to use a clinical decision analysis. B. What are the results and will they help me in caring for my patients? JAMA 1995; 273: 1610–3.

REPORTS OF ECONOMIC ANALYSES

Sometimes our search for an answer to a therapeutic or other clinical question will yield an economic analysis that compares the costs and consequences of different management decisions. We warn you at the outset that economic analyses are difficult to interpret and often controversial (even among health economists!) and we won't pretend to describe all their nuances here (if you are interested in understanding them, we've suggested some additional resources at the end of this section). Unfortunately, when viewed from the perspective of the evidence-based journals, the number of economic analyses that are judged to be both valid and clinically important is declining.**** They are very demanding for their

---

**** Despite pleas to health economist colleagues to nominate sound and relevant papers, the number of economic analyses published in *Evidence-Based Medicine* fell from 12 in 1996 to 11 in 1997 and five in 1998.

executors, and for us readers as well. For example, they teach us to stop thinking about the costs of a new treatment in terms of pounds and pence/dollars and cents, and to start thinking about them in terms of the other things we can't do if we use our scarce resources to fund this new treatment. This "cost as sacrifice" is better known as "opportunity cost" and is a useful way of thinking in everyday practice, for when we internists "borrow" a bed from our surgical colleagues in order to admit a medical emergency tonight, the opportunity cost of our decision includes canceling tomorrow's elective surgery on the patient for whom the bed was reserved.

These papers are pretty tough to read and you might want to confine your initial searches to the evidence-based journals (such as *ACP Journal Club*, *Evidence-Based Mental Health*, and the like), which not only provide a standard, clear format for reporting economic analyses but also provide expert commentaries.

The following guides should help you decide whether an economic analysis is valid, important, and useful.

Are the results of this economic analysis valid?

Table 5.18 Guides for deciding whether the results of this economic analysis are valid

1. Is this report asking an economic question:
   - that compares all well-defined courses of action?
   - with a specified point of view from which the costs and outcomes are being viewed?
2. Does this economic analysis cite valid evidence on the efficacy of the alternatives?
3. Does this economic analysis identify all the costs and effects we think it should and select credible and accurate measures for them?
4. Was the type of analysis appropriate for the question posed?
5. Was the robustness of the conclusion tested?

We need to begin by remembering that economic analyses are about choices and must therefore ensure that the study included all the sensible, alternative courses of action (e.g. all three of anticoagulation, antiplatelet therapy and cardioversion for patients with non-valvular atrial fibrillation [NVAF]) rather than just one or two of them. If, for example, we found a report that only described the costs of antiplatelet therapy for patients with NVAF, that's an exercise in accounting, not economic analysis, and it wouldn't help us. A valid economic analysis also has to specify the point of view from which the costs and outcomes are being viewed – for example, a hospital might shy away from in-patient cardioversion in favor of discharging a NVAF patient on anticoagulants that would be paid for from the GP's drug budget, whereas society as a whole would want the most cost-effective approach from an overall point of view. Because economic analyses assume (rather than prove) that the alternative courses of action have highly predictable effects, we need to determine whether they cite and summarize solid evidence on the efficacy of alternatives (the same caution we must remember when reading a CDA). So, was an explicit and sensible process used to identify and appraise the evidence that would satisfy the criteria for validity displayed back in Table 5.1?

All the costs and effects of the treatment should be identified, and credible measures should have been made of all of them. The cost side here can be tricky, since we may want the report to include all the costs of training, housing and sustaining the "whos" and what they do to the "whoms", including all the subsequent costs and consequences of the initial actions. In similar fashion, we need to consider if the investigators have included all outcomes we think are important. Moreover, a high-quality economic analysis should also include (and explain!) discounting future costs and outcomes (to acknowledge the fact that a bird in the hand is worth two in next year's bush).

We need to consider if the type of analysis was appropriate for the question the investigators posed, and this isn't as hard as it sounds. If the question was "Is there a cheaper (but equally effective) way to care for this patient?", the paper should ignore the outcomes and simply compare costs (a "cost minimization" analysis). If the question was "Which way of treating this patient gives the greatest health 'bang for the buck'?", the method of analysis is determined by the sorts of outcomes being compared. If they are identical for all the treatment alternatives (say, whether it's cheaper to prevent embolic stroke in NVAF patients with aspirin or warfarin), and the outcome (stroke) is identical for both treatments, the appropriate analysis is a "cost-effectiveness" analysis. If, however, the outcomes as well as the interventions differ ("Do we get a bigger bang for our buck treating kids for leukemia or their elders for senile dementia?"), the authors will have had to come up with some way of measuring these disparate outcomes with the same yardstick, and there are two of these. First, they could convert both sets of outcomes into their monetary values: a "cost–benefit" analysis. The challenge in cost–benefit analysis is setting these monetary values: should they be earning power (in which case we treat the kids and warehouse their elders) or can we put a value on life itself? No wonder that cost–benefit analysis lacks popularity. The other common yardstick for disparate outcomes is their social (rather than monetary) value: how do patients view their desirability compared with other outcomes (including perfect health and death and the fates worse than death)? A shorthand economic term for this desirability and these preferences is "utility", and utilities can be combined with time to generate "quality-adjusted life-years" (QALYs) (so that 1 year in perfect health is judged equivalent to 3 years in a post-stroke state whose utility is only 0.3). The corresponding economic analysis is called "cost–utility" analysis. So, we need to decide whether the form of economic analysis we find in the paper is appropriate to the question it attempted to answer.

Finally, as when reviewing a clinical decision analysis, we'd like to find a sensitivity analysis. Did the authors examine the impact of inserting clinically sensible differences in costs and effects into their analysis?

If the economic analysis fails the above tests for validity, it's back to searching. If it passes, we can proceed to considering whether its valid results are important.

Are the valid results of this economic analysis important?

Table 5.19 Guides for deciding whether the valid results of this economic analysis are important

1. Are the resulting costs or cost/unit of health gained clinically significant?
2. Did the results of this economic analysis change with sensible changes to costs and effectiveness?

Are the resulting costs or cost/unit of health gained clinically significant? We need to consider whether the intervention will provide a benefit at an acceptable cost. If it is a cost-minimization analysis, we should consider if the difference in cost is big enough to warrant switching to a cheaper one. For a cost-effectiveness analysis, is the difference in effectiveness great enough for us to want to spend the difference? If a cost–utility analysis was done, how do the QALYs generated from spending resources on this treatment compare with those that would result if we spent them in other ways? This comparison is made superficially easier by the growing popularity of cost–utility "league tables". Several league tables have been generated, and we show you one in Table 5.20, with the caution that such tables can both inform and mislead (if their cost and effectiveness data are out of date or inapplicable in your setting).

Table 5.20 A league table of how much it costs to gain one additional quality-adjusted life-year (QALY) for different treatments

Treatment	Cost/QALY (£, August 1990)
Cholesterol testing and diet therapy (all adults aged 40–69)	220
Neurosurgical intervention for head injury	240
Advice to stop smoking from general practitioner	270
Neurosurgical intervention for subarachnoid hemorrhage	490
Antihypertensive treatment to prevent stroke (ages 45–64)	940
Pacemaker implantation	1100
Hip replacement	1180

Table 5.20 *(cont'd)*

Treatment	Cost/QALY (£, August 1990)
Valve replacement for aortic stenosis	1140
Coronary artery bypass graft (left main vessel disease, severe angina)	2090
Kidney transplant	4710
Breast cancer screening	5780
Heart transplantation	7840
Cholesterol testing and treatment (incrementally) of all adults aged 25–39	14 150
Home hemodialysis	17 260
Coronary artery bypass graft (one vessel disease, moderate angina)	18 830
Continuous ambulatory peritoneal dialysis	19 870
Hospital hemodialysis	21 970
Erythropoietin treatment for anemia in dialysis patients (assuming 10% reduction in mortality)	54 380
Neurosurgical intervention for malignant intracranial tumors	107 780
Erythropoietin treatment for anemia in dialysis patients (assuming no increase in survival)	126 290

Adapted from: Mason J, Drummond M, Torrance G. Some guidelines on the use of cost-effectiveness league tables. BMJ 1993; 306: 570–2.

Are the valid, important results of this economic analysis applicable to our patient/practice?

Table 5.21 Guides for deciding whether the valid, important results of this economic analysis are applicable to our patient

1. Do the costs in the economic analysis apply in our setting?
2. Are the treatments likely to be effective in our setting?

As usual, we begin by considering whether our patient is so different from those included in the study that its results are not applicable. We can do this by estimating our patient's probabilities of the various outcomes, and by asking the patient to generate the utilities for these outcomes. If these values fall within the ranges used in the analysis, we can be satisfied that the "effectiveness" results can be applied to our patient. Next we can consider whether the intervention would be used in the same way in our practice.

We then turn to comparing the costs of applying this intervention in the study and carrying it out in our own setting. Costs may be different because of different practice patterns and because local prices for resources vary. If this is so, and if we think they would be different, are our personal cost estimates in the range tested in the sensitivity analysis?

If the paper satisfies all of the above tests, we can celebrate. But if it fails any of them, it's back to the searching process!

Further reading about economic analysis

Drummond M F, Richardson W S, O'Brien B J, Levine M, Heyland D, for the Evidence-Based Medicine Working Group Party. Users' guides to the medical literature: XIII. How to use an article on economic analysis of clinical practice: A. Are the results of the study valid? JAMA 1997; 277: 1552–7.

O'Brien B, Heyland D, Richardson W S, Levine M, Drummond M, for the Evidence-Based Medicine Working Group Party. Users' guides to the medical literature: XIII. How to use an article on economic analysis of clinical practice: B. What are the results and will they help me in caring for my patients? JAMA 1997; 277: 1802–6.

N-OF-1 TRIALS

You may not always be able to find a randomized trial or systematic review relevant to your patient. Traditionally, when faced with this dilemma, we clinicians have conducted a "trial of therapy" during which we start our patient on a treatment and follow him to determine whether the symptoms improve or worsen while on this treatment. Performing this standard trial of therapy may be misleading (and is prone to bias) for several reasons:

1. Some target disorders are self-limited and patients may get better on their own.

2. Both extreme lab values and clinical signs, if left untreated and remeasured later, often return to normal.

3. The placebo effect can lead to substantial improvement in symptoms.

4. Both our own and our patient's expectations about the success or failure of a treatment can bias conclusions about whether a treatment actually works.

5. Polite patients may exaggerate the effects of therapy.

If a treatment is used during any of the above situations, it would tend to appear efficacious when it was useless.

The n-of-1 trial applies the principles of rigorous clinical trial methodology (randomization, blinding, assessment of outcomes) to overcome these problems when trying to determine the best treatment for an individual patient. The n-of-1 randomizes time, and assigns the patient (using concealed randomization and at least single-blinding) to receive active therapy or placebo at different times, so that the resulting multiple crossovers will help both our patient and us to decide on the best therapy. It is employed when there is significant doubt about whether a treatment is helpful, and is most successful when directed toward the control of symptoms or relapses resulting from a chronic disease (e.g. chronic obstructive airways disease).

Guides that we use in deciding whether or not to execute an n-of-1 trial are listed in Table 5.22.

The crucial first step in this process is to have a discussion with the patient to determine his interest, willingness to participate, expectations of the treatment, and desired outcomes. If formal ethics approval is required,[††††] we need to get that process underway at the start.

If, after reviewing these guides, it is decided to do an n-of-1 trial, we use the following tactics (they are described in detail elsewhere):[‡‡‡‡]

[††††] Research ethics approval hasn't been required where we've worked, since the objective here is better care for an individual patient who is a co-investigator.

[‡‡‡‡] Guyatt G, Sackett D, Adachi J, Roberts R, Chong J, Rosenbloom D, Keller J A. A clinician's guide for conducting randomized trials in individual patients. CMAJ 1998; 139: 497–503.

Table 5.22 Guides for n-of-1 randomized trials

1. Is an n-of-1 trial indicated for our patient?
   - Is the effectiveness of the treatment really in doubt for our patient?
   - Will the treatment, if effective, be continued long-term?
   - Is our patient willing and eager to collaborate in designing and carrying out an n-of-1 trial?

2. Is an n-of-1 trial feasible in our patient?
   - Does the treatment have a rapid onset?
   - Does the treatment cease to act soon after it is discontinued?
   - Is the optimal treatment duration feasible?
   - Can outcomes that are relevant and important to our patient be measured?
   - Can we establish sensible criteria for stopping the trial?
   - Can an unblinded run-in period be conducted?

3. Is an n-of-1 trial feasible in our practice setting?
   - Is there a pharmacist available to help?
   - Are strategies for interpreting the trial data in place?

4. Is the n-of-1 study ethical?
   - Is approval by our medical research ethics committee necessary?

1. We agree on the symptoms, signs or other manifestations of our patient's target disorder that we want to improve, and set up a diary so that our patient can record them at regular intervals.

2. We agree (in collaboration with a pharmacist) on the active and comparison (usually placebo) treatments, treatment durations, and rules for stopping a treatment period.

3. Our patient then undergoes pairs of treatment periods in which he receives the experimental therapy during one period and the placebo during the other, the order of active or placebo treatment being randomized.

4. If possible, both we and our patient remain blind to the treatment being given during any period, even when we examine the results at the end of the pair of periods.

5. Pairs of treatment periods are replicated and analyzed until one or both of us decides to unblind the results and decide whether to continue the active therapy or abandon it.

Further reading about n-of-1 trials

Guyatt G, Sackett D, Adachi J, Roberts R, Chong J, Rosenbloom D, Keller J A. A clinician's guide for conducting randomized trials in individual patients. CMAJ 1998; 139: 497–503.

Guyatt G H, Keller J L, Jaeschke R, Rosenbloom D, Adachi J D, Newhouse M T. The n-of-1 randomized controlled trial: clinical usefulness. Our three-year experience. Ann Intern Med 1990; 112: 293–9.

Sackett D L, Haynes R B, Guyatt G H, Tugwell P. Clinical epidemiology: a basic science for clinical medicine, 2nd edn. Little, Brown, Boston, 1991.

Harm

We frequently must make judgements about whether a medical intervention or an environmental agent is harming our patient. Questions such as "Do oral contraceptives cause breast cancer?" or "Do calcium antagonists increase the risk of death or cancer?" are being posed by both us and our patients. One of us even had a patient come to our clinic with headlines from newspaper stories pulled off the internet claiming: "Hypertension med kills!" We'll use his (and our!) dilemma as the ongoing example in this chapter.

To answer questions about harm, we need to be able to evaluate evidence about causation for its validity, importance and direct relevance to our patients. Assessing the validity of the evidence is crucial if we are to avoid drawing the false-positive conclusion that an agent does cause an adverse event when, in truth, it does not; or the false-negative conclusion that an agent does not cause an adverse event when, in truth, it does. Even clinical pharmacologists disagree about whether a given patient has had an adverse drug reaction – and just because an adverse event occurred during treatment, it does not inevitably follow that the adverse event occurred because of that treatment.

ARE THE RESULTS OF THIS HARM/AETIOLOGY STUDY VALID?

This chapter begins with guides that we can use to assess the validity of studies about harm, shown in Table 6.1. We'll use the above patient's dilemma to ask the clinical question "Are patients taking calcium antagonists at increased risk of developing cancer?" in order to explore these guides in detail.

The "threats to validity" are different for different study types, and this affects our search. In considering whether exposure to calcium antagonists causes cancer, we've learned that systematic reviews of all relevant studies constitute the highest

6

Table 6.1 Is this evidence about harm valid?

1. Were there clearly defined groups of patients, similar in all important ways other than exposure to the treatment or other cause?

2. Were treatments/exposures and clinical outcomes measured in the same ways in both groups? (Was the assessment of outcomes either objective or blinded to exposure?)

3. Was the follow-up of the study patients sufficiently long (for the outcome to occur and complete)?

4. Do the results of the harm study fulfil some of the diagnostic tests for causation?

   - Is it clear that the exposure preceded the onset of the outcome?
   - Is there a dose–response gradient?
   - Is there any positive evidence from a "dechallenge–rechallenge" study?
   - Is the association consistent from study to study?
   - Does the association make biological sense?

level of evidence, so these should always be our primary targets in any search. Individual randomized trials are seldom of sufficient size to detect rare adverse events with precision, which is all the more reason to look for systematic reviews of multiple randomized trials or cohort studies, where we might find sufficiently large numbers of patients to identify even rare adverse effects. As with any systematic review, we need to assess it twice for validity, once using the guides in Table 6.1 and again using the guides for systematic reviews presented in Chapter 5 (Table 5.9).

1. Were there clearly defined groups of patients, similar in all important ways other than exposure to the treatment or other cause?

Ideally our search would unearth a systematic review or a randomized trial in which patients with hypertension had been allocated, by a system analogous to tossing a coin, to receive a calcium antagonist (the top row in Table 6.2, whose total is $a + b$), or some comparison treatment or placebo (the bottom row in Table 6.2, whose total is $c + d$).

Randomization would tend to make the two treatment groups identical for all other causes of cancer, so we'd likely consider any statistically significant increase in cancers in the calcium

Table 6.2 Studies of whether calcium antagonists cause cancer

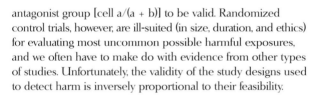

		Adverse outcome (cancer)		Totals
		Present (case)	Absent (control)	
Exposed to the treatment (calcium antagonist)	Yes (RCT or cohort)	a	b	a+b
	No (RCT or cohort)	c	d	c+d
	Totals	a+c	b+d	a+b+c+d

antagonist group [cell a/(a + b)] to be valid. Randomized control trials, however, are ill-suited (in size, duration, and ethics) for evaluating most uncommon possible harmful exposures, and we often have to make do with evidence from other types of studies. Unfortunately, the validity of the study designs used to detect harm is inversely proportional to their feasibility.

In the first of these alternatives, a cohort study, groups of patients (cohorts) who are (a + b) and are not (c + d) exposed to the treatment are followed for the development of the outcome of interest (a or c). Using the searching strategies outlined in Chapter 2, we found an article describing a cohort study that looked at the association between the use of calcium antagonists and the risk of cancer.* This study assembled cancer-free cohorts 71 years of age or older from three regions in the US who were (a + b) and weren't (c + d) taking calcium antagonists. These cohorts were clearly defined but heterogeneous, as more of the exposed group had diabetes, cardiovascular disease, disability and hospital admissions.

Because the decision to prescribe and accept exposure is purposive, not randomized, in a cohort study "exposed" patients may differ from "non-exposed" patients for important determinants of the outcome (such determinants are called confounders).[†] Considering a hypothetical example, if people with hypertension were more likely to develop cancer than normotensives, hypertension would be a confounder when comparing the risk of cancer in people using and not using calcium antagonists (or any other antihypertensive drug). Investigators must document the characteristics of both cohorts of patients and either demonstrate their comparability or adjust for the confounders they identify. Of course, they can only adjust for confounders that are already known and have been measured, so we have to be careful when interpreting cohort studies.[‡]

If the outcome of interest is rare or takes a long time to develop, even large cohort studies may not be feasible and we will have to look to case–control studies. In this study design, people with the outcome of interest (a + c) are identified as "cases" and those without it (b + d) are selected as controls and the proportion of each group who were exposed to the putative agent (a or b) is assessed retrospectively. There is even more potential for confounding with case–control studies than with cohort studies because confounders that are transient or lead to early death won't even be able to be measured. For example, if patients are selected from hospital sources, the relationship between outcome and exposure will be distorted if patients who are exposed are more likely to be admitted to the hospital than are the unexposed. This was illustrated nicely in a recent systematic review which looked at the association between vasectomy and prostate cancer. The relative risk of prostate cancer following vasectomy was elevated in hospital-based studies but not in population-based ones.

It is also important that the control patients should have the same opportunity for exposure to the putative agent. If we found a case–control study of calcium antagonists and cancer that assembled cancer patients as the cases but excluded patients with coronary artery disease (who are at increased risk

---

[†] These determinants are called confounders when they have the three properties of being: extraneous to the questions posed, determinants of the outcomes, and unequally distributed between exposed and non-exposed study patients.

[‡] That's another great thing about randomization; it balances groups for unknown confounders we haven't yet discovered.

of exposure) from the control group, we'd be right to wonder whether an observed association was spurious.

Finally, we may only find case reports of one or a few patients who developed an adverse event while receiving the suspected treatment (cell a). If the outcome is unusual and dramatic enough (phocomelia in children born to women who took thalidomide), such case reports and case series may be enough to answer our question. But because these studies lack comparison groups, they are usually only sufficient for hypothesis generation and thus point to the need for other studies.

2. Were treatments/exposures and clinical outcomes measured in the same ways in both groups? (Was the assessment of outcomes either objective or blinded to exposure?)

We should place greater confidence in studies in which treatment exposures and clinical outcomes were measured in the same way in both groups. If, for example, a report examined the use of calcium antagonists and the risk of cancer, we'd be concerned if it indicated that the investigator searched more aggressively for cancer in the patients who were known to use calcium antagonists. Similarly, patients with the adverse event may be more likely to have brooded about their sad situation and may have greater ability or incentive to recall possible exposure. Thus, we'd feel more assured about the study if the report described that the patients (and their interviewers!) were blinded to the study hypothesis. In the study that we found to answer our question, participants were asked to show all containers for all prescription and non-prescription drugs taken over the previous 2 weeks. Hospital discharge information, the national death registry and a cancer registry were used to determine the occurrence of new cancers. We reckoned that both of these features added to the credibility of this report.

3. Was the follow-up of the study patients sufficiently long (for the outcome to occur) and complete?

If we found a study of the association between calcium antagonists and cancer that followed patients for only a few weeks, we couldn't distinguish a true- from a false-negative association (in the study we found, a mean follow-up of 3.7 years yielded only 47 cancers from 1549 person-years of taking calcium antagonists).

Similarly, if the study lost lots of its patients to follow-up (>20% is a good rule of thumb), we'd also be skeptical of its conclusions, because lost patients may have very different outcomes from those who remain in the study.

4. Do the results of the harm study fulfil some of the diagnostic tests for causation?

Is it clear that the exposure preceded the onset of the outcome? We'd want to make sure that the exposure (e.g. to the calcium antagonist) occurred prior to the development of the adverse outcome (e.g. cancer) and wasn't just a marker that it was already underway. In our study, all patients known to have cancer at the beginning of the study were excluded.

Is there a dose–response gradient? The demonstration of an increasing risk (or severity) of the adverse event with increasing exposure (increased dose and/or duration) to the putative causal agent strengthens the association. In the calcium antagonist–cancer study there was a dose–response gradient.

Is there any positive evidence from a "dechallenge–rechallenge" study? This occurs when the adverse outcome decreases or disappears when the treatment is withdrawn and worsens or reappears when it is reintroduced. Returning to our clinical scenario, cancer usually persists and therefore this guide doesn't apply.

Is the association consistent from study to study? If we were able to find multiple studies or, better yet, a systematic review of the question, we could determine whether the association between exposure and the adverse event is consistent from study to study. For our question, there have been several case–control and cohort studies of death following calcium antagonists, some finding an association and others not.

Does the association make biological sense? If the association between exposure and outcome makes biological sense (in terms of pathophysiology, etc.), a causal interpretation becomes more plausible. In our example, the authors offered interference with apoptosis as a possible mechanism for the association between calcium antagonists and cancer. However, as this edition went to press, apoptosis was the "hypothesis du jour" for investigators trying to explain results and was being hotly debated.

ARE THE VALID RESULTS OF THIS HARM STUDY IMPORTANT?

If the study we find fails to satisfy the first three minimum standards in Table 6.1, we'd probably be better off abandoning it and continuing our search. But if we are satisfied that it meets these minimum guides, we need to decide if the association between exposure and outcome is sufficiently strong and convincing for us to have to do something about it. By this, we mean looking at the risk or odds of the adverse effect with (as opposed to without) exposure to the treatment; the higher the risk or odds, the stronger the association and the more we should be impressed by it. We can use the single guide in Table 6.3 to determine if the valid results of the study are important.

1. What is the magnitude and precision of the association between the exposure and outcome?

Different study architectures require different methods for estimating the strength of association between exposure to the putative cause and the outcome of interest. For randomized trials and cohort studies, the most common way of describing the results is by calculating the incidence (in this situation we call it the "risk") of the adverse event in the treated patients relative to the risk in the untreated patients: $[a/(a + b)]/[c/(c + d)]$ (from Table 6.2). For example, if 1000 patients receive a treatment and 20 of them have an adverse

Table 6.3 Are the valid results of this harm study important?

1. What is the magnitude and precision of the association between the exposure and outcome?

outcome, a = 20 and a/(a + b) = 2%. If just 2 of 1000 patients who do not receive this treatment for the same target disorder experienced this adverse event, c = 2 and c/(c + d) = 2/1000 = 0.2% and the relative risk = 2%/0.2% = 10. This means that patients receiving the suspect treatment are 10 times as likely to suffer the adverse event as patients treated the other way.

Because case–control studies sample outcomes rather than exposures, we can't calculate "incidences" such as relative risks from them. Rather, the strength of association in a case–control study can only be indirectly estimated and is presented as an odds ratio (or relative odds): ad/bc. If, for example, 100 cases of the adverse outcome are identified and it is found that 90 of them had received the putative causal agent, a = 90 and c = 10. If 100 control patients (free of the adverse outcome) are assembled and it is discovered that 45 of them received the suspect treatment, b = 45 and d = 55 and the relative odds = ad/bc = (90 × 55)/(45 × 10) = 11. This means that the odds of experiencing the adverse event for patients exposed to the putative causal agent is 11 times that of those patients not receiving it.

How big should relative risks and odds ratios be before we should be impressed with them? This brings us back a bit into issues of validity. Odds ratios (ORs) and relative risks (RRs) greater than 1 indicate that there is an increased risk of the adverse outcome associated with the exposure (we hope it is sensible to you that when the RR or OR = 1, the adverse outcome is no more likely to occur with than without exposure to the suspected agent). Because cohort studies and, even more so, case–control studies are susceptible to many biases,[§] we want to ensure that the OR is greater than that which could result from bias alone. In a recent personal communication, Professor Richard Doll reported that "It's almost impossible to set a level of risk which is so high that findings in a well-conducted epidemiological study would necessarily exclude confounding. I am on record as having said that 20-fold excesses are in themselves almost sufficient to indicate causality!"** We might not want to label an odds ratio from a case–control study as impressive unless it is greater than 4 for minor adverse events and set this value at progressively lower levels as the severity of the adverse event increases. There is less potential bias in cohort studies and therefore we might regard a relative risk of greater than 3 as convincing for more severe adverse events. In the cohort study of calcium antagonists and cancer we unearthed, the relative risk was an unimpressive 1.4.

On the other hand, Professor Irwig has suggested a sensitivity analysis for determining whether an odds ratio or relative risk is impressive.†† It can be carried out on a report that includes at least some "adjustment" or "correction" for potential confounders. He suggests comparing the unadjusted measure of association with one in which at least one known confounder has been adjusted out: if this adjustment produces a large decline in RR or OR, we should be suspicious of both of them. If, in contrast, the adjusted RR or OR is stable with this adjustment, or if it rises rather than falls, our confidence in the validity of the association would be greater. In the study we found, the RR rose from 1.4 to 1.7 when it was adjusted for several differences in patients' baseline characteristics, suggesting that confounding (of cancer risk and calcium antagonist use) did not explain the results.

In addition to looking at the magnitude of the RR or OR, we need to look at its precision by examining the confidence interval around it. Credibility is highest when the entire confidence interval is narrow and remains within a clinically importantly increased risk (in our study, the 95% confidence interval is 1.27–2.34 which is statistically significant).

Although the OR and RR tell us about the strength of the association, we need to translate this into some measure that is useful and intelligible both to us and our patient. For this, we can turn to the number needed to harm (NNH), which tells us the "number of patients who need to be exposed to

---

** Personal communication to the authors from Professor Doll, December 1997.

†† Personal communication to the authors from Professor Irwig, November 1997.

the putative causal agent to produce one additional harmful event". The NNH can be calculated directly from trials and cohort studies in a fashion analogous to the NNT, but this time as the reciprocal of the difference in adverse event rates = $[a/(a + b)] - [c/(c + d)]$. For an OR derived from a case–control study, the calculation is more complex (remember, we can't determine "incidence" directly in a case–control study). Its scary formula reads:

$$1 - [PEER \times (1 - OR)]/(1 - PEER) \times PEER \times (1 - OR)$$

where PEER is the patient expected event rate (the adverse event rate among individuals who are not exposed to the putative cause). We've made this easier for you by cranking out some typical PEERs and ORs and summarizing them in Table 6.4.

Table 6.4 NNHs derived from typical PEERs and ORs[a]

		For odds ratios LESS than 1						
		0.9	0.8	0.7	0.6	0.5	0.4	0.3
	0.05	209	104	69	52	41	34	29
Patient	0.10	110	54	36	27	21	18	15
expected	0.20	61	30	20	14	11	10	8
event	0.30	46	22	14	10	8	7	5
rate	0.40	40	19	12	9	7	6	4
(PEER)	0.50	38	18	11	8	6	5	4
	0.70	44	20	13	9	6	5	4
	0.90	101	46	27	18	12	9	4
		For odds ratios GREATER than 1						
		1.1	1.25	1.5	1.75	2	2.25	2.5
	0.05	212	86	44	30	23	18	16
Patient	0.10	113	46	24	16	13	10	9
expected	0.20	64	27	14	10	8	7	6
event	0.30	50	21	11	8	7	6	5
rate	0.40	44	19	10	8	6	5	5
(PEER)	0.50	42	18	10	8	6	6	5
	0.70	51	23	13	10	9	8	7
	0.90	121	55	33	25	22	19	18

[a] Adapted from John Geddes, 1999.

As you can see from the table, for different PEERs, the same OR can lead to very different NNHs and it is therefore important that we do your best to estimate our patient's expected event rate when calculating the NNH. For example, if the OR is 0.90 and the PEER was 0.005, the NNH would be 2000, but if the PEER was 0.40, the NNH would be 40. We'll consider individual patients more in the next section. Once we have decided that the evidence we have found is both valid and important, we need to consider if it can be applied to our patient (Table 6.5).

CAN THIS VALID AND IMPORTANT EVIDENCE ABOUT HARM BE APPLIED TO OUR PATIENT?

Table 6.5 Guides for deciding whether valid important evidence about harm can be applied to our patient

1. Is our patient so different from those included in the study that its results don't apply?
2. What is our patient's risk of the adverse event? What is our patient's potential benefit from the therapy?
3. What are our patient's preferences, concerns and expectations from this treatment?
4. What alternative treatments are available?

1. Is our patient so different from those included in the study that its results don't apply

As emphasized in previous chapters, the issue is not whether our patient fulfils all the inclusion criteria for the study we found, but whether our patient is so different from those in the study that its results are of no help to us.

2. What is our patient's risk of the adverse event? What is our patient's potential benefit from the therapy?

To apply the results of a study to an individual patient, we need to estimate our patient's risk of the adverse event if he were not exposed to the putative cause. This can be done the hard way by searching for good evidence on prognosis, or the much easier way of estimating the risk relative to that of unexposed individuals in the study. Just as with NNTs in

Chapter 5, we can express this as a decimal fraction (called "f"): if our patient is at half the risk of study patients, $f = 0.5$; if our patient is at three times the risk, $f = 3$. The study NNH can then be divided by f to produce the NNH for our individual patient. For example, the NNH from the study we found is 116, but if we think our patient is at twice the risk of the study patients, $f = 2$ and $116/2$ generates an NNH of 58. If, on the other hand, we thought our patient was at one-third the risk ($f = 0.33$), the NNH for patients like ours becomes 348.

This NNH needs to be balanced against the corresponding NNT summarizing the benefit of this treatment. The resulting crude "likelihood of being helped vs. harmed" (LHH, see Ch. 5) by this treatment can provide the starting point for the last step, described in the next section.

3. What are our patient's preferences, concerns and expectations from this treatment?

It is vital that we incorporate our patient's unique concerns and preferences into any shared decision-making process. In the case of potentially harmful therapy, and just as in Chapter 5, we can ask our patient to quantify his values for both the potential adverse event and the target event we hope to prevent with the proposed therapy. The result is a severity-adjusted likelihood of being helped or harmed by the therapy. If we are unsure of our patient's baseline risk, or if he is unsure about his values for the outcomes, a sensitivity analysis can be done. That is, different values for relative severity could be inserted and we and our patient could determine at which point the decision would change.

4. What alternative treatments are available?

Finally, we and our patient could explore alternative management options. In the example we have been considering, there is a wide array of alternative treatments available for hypertension (thiazides and beta-blockers) that have been found to be effective in high-quality studies, and while they do have side-effects, these are not reputed to cause cancer. We discussed these alternative treatments with our patient and his GP so that they could decide on his long-term management.

A FINAL NOTE

This chapter has been written to assist deliberations about whether treatments do more harm than good, for this is the typical perspective of hospital-based internists. Other readers may be more likely to consider questions of causation around lifestyle issues such as cigarette smoking, diet, and exercise. The principles are all the same, but in lifestyle issues, the harm is contrasted with the satisfaction or other gains derived from pursuing the "unhealthy" practice. To provide readers with this latter perspective, we'll install a lifestyle issue on this book's website: <http://www.library.utoronto.ca/medicine/ebm/>.

MAKING A SUMMARY

Now that we've gone to all the effort of retrieving an article and critically appraising it, it would be nice to keep a summary of it so that we (and others) can refer to it in the future. We've enclosed a CAT (see Ch. 3) for the calcium antagonist article that we found.

Further reading

Levine M, Walter S D, Lee H, Haines T, Holbrook A, Moyer V for the Evidence-Based Medicine Working Group. Users' guides to the medical literature. IV. How to use an article about harm. JAMA 1994; 271: 1615–19.

Sackett D L, Haynes R B, Guyatt G H, Tugwell P. Clinical epidemiology. A basic science for clinical medicine, 2nd edn. Little, Brown, Boston, 1991.

Straus S E, Sackett D L, Bates S M, Rekers H, Ginsberg J S. Levels of evidence for evaluating clinical literature about harm/aetiology. In press.

CAT Hypertension – calcium-channel blockers may cause cancer

Clinical bottom line(s)
1. Until this gets sorted out properly, if your patient's problem could be treated as well by some alternative drug (e.g. hypertension), it would be prudent to avoid using calcium-channel agents.
2. If this result is true, the NNH to cause one additional cancer from taking CCBs for 3.7 years is 116.

Citation. Pahor M et al. Calcium-channel blockade and incidence of cancer in aged populations. Lancet 1996; 348: 493–7 (also see 487–9 and 541–2).

Clinical question. Are patients taking calcium antagonists for hypertension at increased risk of cancer?

Search terms: from the newspaper headline or from MEDLINE using "calcium antagonists" and "cancer".

The study
Total or stratified random samples (>80% response rate) of 65+ y/o men and women in three sites in the USA. Showed their meds, were interviewed for 90 minutes, and had their blood pressure, height and weight measured. Anyone with cancer in previous 3 years or on any cancer Rx was excluded and 94% of the remainder were followed for an average of 3.7 years by follow-up interview, hospital discharge information and the national death registry for the occurrence of new cancers.

The evidence

		Later cancer		Totals
		Present	Absent	
Exposed to calcium-channel blockers	Yes (cohort)	3.03% a	b	a+b
	No (cohort)	c 2.17%	d	c+d
	Totals	a+c	b+d	a+b+c+d

Relative risk (RR) = 3.03%/2.17% = 1.4 ($P = 0.032$) (and when adjusted for several baseline differences, RR *rose* (!) to 1.7 ($P = 0.0005$)).

Comments
1. Individuals on CCBs had more cardiovascular disease, diabetes, disability, and hospitalizations but lower diastolic blood pressure. But when they adjusted for all these baseline differences, the RR rose rather than fell, suggesting that bias from confounding (of cancer risk and CCB use) of these characteristics could not explain these results.
2. There was a dose–response gradient.
3. The difference in risk by type of CCB was impressive but not statistically significant (RR = 2 for verapamil; 1.5 for nifedipine; 0.94 for diltiazem).
4. Only 47 events in CCB takers, and spread over all sorts of different cancers.
5. The proposed mechanism (interference with the apoptotic destruction of cancer cells) has been pooh-poohed by commentators.
6. Other studies of CCBs and mortality go both ways (they're bad or have no effect), and some authors of the former have received anonymous death threats.

Appraised by: Sackett, 1996.   *Expiry date:* 2001.

Guidelines

Most clinicians develop "routines" for the evaluation and management of the illnesses we frequently encounter. For example, when faced with a patient with clinically suspected acute myocardial infarction, the authors of this book can reel off the "appropriate" pre-hospital evaluation and management (quick exam, ambulance, aspirin, and analgesia), immediate hospital care (stat and serial exams, EKGs, enzymes, blood sugar, electrolytes and, if appropriate, fibrinolytics, beta-blockers, ACE inhibitors, and an insulin–glucose infusion), pre-discharge discussions with the patient, the family and the GP (about follow-up investigations, smoking, long-term beta-blockers and aspirin and ACE inhibitors, lipid-lowering, other risk factors, exercise, sex, and return to full activity), and long-term care.

Where do these routines come from? For us, their first drafts were generated as postgraduate trainees and resulted from "replicating" the advice of our respected teachers and/or the commands of our consultants (not necessarily the same people!). Later, as we gained the ability and freedom to operate in the "searching" and "appraising" modes, they were added to (statins), subtracted from (prophylactic lidocaine) and modified on the basis of the highest quality evidence we could find, tempered by our patients' values and the local conditions in which we worked. This process of repeatedly searching, appraising, and modifying our management routines costs us lots of time and energy, but because we encounter such patients daily, we consider the effort well spent.

But what about the conditions we see less often (e.g. Guillain–Barré syndrome, temporal arteritis, or carbon monoxide poisoning)? When faced with these less common problems, we shift to the "searching" mode we described back in the Introduction, restrict our quest to high-quality, previously appraised evidence (such as that provided by the Cochrane Library and the evidence-based journals) or might

7

even see whether we can quickly find a relevant battery of "systematically developed statements to assist practitioner and patient decisions about appropriate health care for specific clinical circumstances".[1]* As it happens, some thoughtful colleagues have named such statements "guidelines", and majuscular amounts of time and money (alas, often with unnecessary duplication) are currently being invested in their production, application, and evaluation. This very brief chapter is designed to help busy clinicians decide both whether a guideline is worth using and whether one is worth writing. Readers who want to learn more than this about them should look elsewhere.[2]

In a nutshell, if we're considering using a guideline, we should think of it as having two distinct components, as depicted in Table 7.1: first, the evidence summary ("here's the average effect of this intervention on the typical patient who accepts it") and second, the detailed instructions for applying that evidence to our patient. Then we should look at the two components individually. We apply our eye and nose to the first component, the evidence summary: our eye, to see if it tracked down all the relevant evidence and graded it for its validity; and our nose, to smell whether it has updated its review recently enough to still be fresh. Then we apply our ear to the second component to listen for any "killer Bs"† in our neighborhood that would make its detailed instructions impossible to execute. And if we're asked to (help) write one, we should never volunteer to labor in the first component (except as a member of a Cochrane Review Group), but insist that we be appointed to the second component as the local "B-keeper".

Although valid guidelines create their evidence components from systematic reviews of all the relevant worldwide literature,

---

* And if we can't find any, we slip into the "replicating" mode and holler for help from the nearest expert.

† These are: an insufficient *B*urden to warrant action; strong *B*eliefs that the risks of the recommended maneuvers outweigh their benefits; other, better *B*argains for the use of your resources; and insurmountable *B*arriers to their adoption. Thanks to Andy Oxman for helping us name and characterize them. We'll explain them fully in the paragraphs introduced by Table 7.4.

Table 7.1 The two distinct components of any guideline

	The evidence component	The detailed instructional component
Bottom line	"Here's the typical effect of this diagnostic/ therapeutic/preventive intervention on the typical patient"	"Here is exactly what to do to/ with this patient"
Underlying requirements	Validity Importance Up-to-datedness	Local relevance
Expertise required by those executing this component	Human biology, clinical science, consumerism, database searching, clinical epidemiology, biostatistics	Clinical practice, local patient values, local current practice, local geography, local economics, local sociology, local politics, local tradition
Site where this component should be generated	National or international	Local
Form of output	Levels of evidence	Grades of recommendations and detailed instructions, flow charts, protocols (perhaps computer-driven)

there's an important distinction between them and the "free-standing" reviews we encounter in the clinical journals. The free-standing systematic reviews you first met back in Chapter 2 tend to be "evidence-driven" and are likely to appear only when there is high-quality evidence (even Cochrane Reviews are usually restricted to randomized trials). By contrast, the reviews that provide the evidence components for guidelines are "necessity-driven" and synthesize the best evidence (even if it is of shaky quality) that can be found to guide an urgent decision that has to be made tonight. It necessarily follows that some recommendations in the second component of a guideline may be derived from evidence of high validity and others from evidence that is much more liable to error. Accordingly, it is important that these different "levels" of evidence are acknowledged in tying the evidence to the clinical recommendations. This need was recognized back in the 1970s by the Canadian Task Force on the Periodic Health Exam,[3] and ever more sophisticated ways of describing and categorizing levels of evidence have followed.[4] In the present era, they have been an important element of at least some of the clinical texts on "evidence-based practice" in which each clinical recommendation is accompanied by an icon denoting the level of evidence that was employed in generating it. Table 7.2 lists the levels used by an energetic group of doctors-in-training in writing the recent and revolutionary house officers' manual: *Evidence-based On-call*.[5] Each of their recommendations is "tagged" with the level of evidence on which it is based.

IS THIS GUIDELINE VALID?

Quite extensive users' guides for deciding on the validity of the evidence components of guidelines have been published,[6,7] but we'll stick to the bare bones shown in Table 7.3.

First, did its developers carry out a comprehensive, reproducible literature review within the past 12 months? Given the problems of "publication bias" we told you about in Chapter 5, a comprehensive review needs to include all relevant articles in all relevant languages (e.g. some of the most important evidence for guidelines about family supports for schizophrenics was published in Mandarin). The 12-month limit is arbitrary and should be shortened for guidelines based on fast-changing evidence and lengthened for the stagnant ones. Second, is each of its recommendations both tagged by the level of evidence upon which it is based and linked to a specific citation? Only in this way can we separate the really solid recommendations from the tenuous ones, and (if we want to appraise the evidence for ourselves) track them back to their sources. As you can see, satisfying these validity guides is a formidable task, and its successful execution requires a combination of clinical, informational, and methodological skills, plus lots of time and money. For this reason, this first

Table 7.2 Levels of evidence and grades of recommendations[a–c]

Grade of recommendation	Level of evidence	Therapy/prevention, aetiology/harm	Prognosis	Diagnosis	Economic analysis
A	1a	SR (with homogeneity[d]) of RCTs	SR (with homogeneity[d]) of inception cohort studies; or a CPG[e] validated on a test set	SR (with homogeneity[d]) of level 1 diagnostic studies; or a CPG validated on a test set	SR (with homogeneity[d]) of level 1 economic studies
	1b	Individual RCT (with narrow confidence interval[f])	Individual inception cohort study with ≥ 80% follow-up	Independent blind comparison of an appropriate spectrum of consecutive patients, all of whom have undergone both the diagnostic test and the reference standard	Analysis comparing all (critically validated) alternative outcomes against appropriate cost measurement, and including a sensitivity analysis incorporating clinically sensible variations in important variables
	1c	All or none[g]	All-or-none case series[h]	Absolute SpPins and SnNouts[i]	Clearly as good or better[j] but cheaper. Clearly as bad or worse but more expensive. Clearly better or worse at the same cost

Table 7.2 (cont'd)

Grade of recommendation	Level of evidence	Therapy/prevention, aetiology/harm	Prognosis	Diagnosis	Economic analysis
	2a	SR (with homogeneity[a]) of cohort studies	SR (with homogeneity[a]) of either retrospective cohort studies or untreated control groups in RCTs	SR (with homogeneity[a]) of level ≥ 2 diagnostic studies	SR (with homogeneity[a]) of level ≥ 2 economic studies
B	2b	Individual cohort study (including low-quality RCT; e.g. <80% follow-up)	Retrospective cohort study or follow-up of untreated control patients in an RCT; or CPG not validated in a test set	Independent blind comparison but either in non-consecutive patients, or confined to a narrow spectrum of study individuals (or both), all of whom have undergone both the diagnostic test and the reference standard; or a diagnostic CPG not validated in a test set	Analysis comparing a limited number of alternative outcomes against appropriate cost measurement, and including a sensitivity analysis incorporating clinically sensible variations in important variables
	2c	"Outcomes" research	"Outcomes" research		

Table 7.2 *(cont'd)*

	3a	SR (with homogeneity^a) of case–control studies			
	3b	Individual case–control study		Independent blind comparison of an appropriate spectrum, but the reference standard was not applied to all study patients	Analysis without accurate cost measurement, but including a sensitivity analysis incorporating clinically sensible variations in important variables
C	4	Case series (and poor-quality cohort and case–control studies^c)	Case series (and poor-quality prognostic cohort studies)	Reference standard was not applied independently or not applied blindly	Analysis with no sensitivity analysis
D	5	Expert opinion without explicit critical appraisal, or based on physiology, bench research or "first principles"	Expert opinion without explicit critical appraisal, or based on physiology, bench research or "first principles"	Expert opinion without explicit critical appraisal, or based on physiology, bench research or "first principles"	Expert opinion without explicit critical appraisal, or based on economic theory

Table 72 (cont'd)

[a] These levels were generated in a series of iterations among members of the NHS R&D Centre for Evidence-Based Medicine (Chris Ball, Dave Sackett, Bob Phillips, Brian Haynes, and Sharon Straus).

[b] Recommendations based on this approach apply to "average" patients and may need to be modified in light of an individual patient's unique biology (risk, responsiveness, etc.) and preferences about the care he or she receives.

[c] Users can add a minus sign (−) to denote the level that fails to provide a conclusive answer because of: *either* a single result with a wide confidence interval (such that, for example, an ARR in an RCT is not statistically significant but whose confidence intervals fail to exclude clinically important benefit or harm); *or* an SR with troublesome (and statistically significant) heterogeneity. Such evidence is inconclusive, and therefore can only generate grade D recommendations.

[d] By homogeneity we mean a systematic review that is free of worrisome variations (heterogeneity) in the directions and degrees of results between individual studies. Not all systematic reviews with statistically significant heterogeneity need be worrisome, and not all worrisome heterogeneity need be statistically significant. As noted above, studies displaying worrisome heterogeneity should be tagged with a "−" at the end of their designated level.

[e] CPG, clinical prediction guide.

[f] See note "c" for advice on how to understand, rate and use trials or other studies with wide confidence intervals.

[g] Met when *all* patients died before the Rx became available, but some now survive on it; or when some patients died before the Rx became available, but *none* now die on it.

[h] Met when there are no reports of anyone with this condition ever avoiding (all or suffering from (none) a particular outcome (such as death).

Table 7.2 (cont'd)

i An "absolute SpPin" is a diagnostic finding whose **Specificity** is so high that a **Positive** result rules **in** the diagnosis. An "absolute SnNout" is a diagnostic finding whose **Sensitivity** is so high that a **Negative** result rules **out** the diagnosis.

j Good, better, bad, and worse refer to the comparisons between treatments in terms of their clinical risks and benefits.

k By poor-quality *cohort study*, we mean one that failed to clearly define comparison groups and/or failed to measure exposures and outcomes in the same (preferably blinded) objective way in both exposed and non-exposed individuals and/or failed to identify or appropriately control known confounders and/or failed to carry out a sufficiently long and complete follow-up of patients. By poor quality *case–control study*, we mean one that failed to clearly define comparison groups and/or failed to measure exposures and outcomes in the same blinded, objective way in both cases and controls and/or failed to identify or appropriately control known cofounders.

l By poor-quality prognostic cohort study, we mean one in which sampling was biased in favor of patients who already had the target outcome, or the measurement of outcomes was accomplished in < 80% of study patients, or outcomes were determined in an unblinded, non-objective way, or there was no correction for confounding factors.

Table 7.3 Guides for deciding whether a guideline is valid

1. Did its developers carry out a comprehensive, reproducible literature review within the past 12 months?

2. Is each of its recommendations both tagged by the level of evidence upon which it is based and linked to a specific citation?

component of guideline development is best filled by a national or international collaboration of sufficient scope and size to not only carry out the systematic review but to update it as often as important new evidence appears on the scene. If a guideline fails one or both of these guides, we can't tell whether its application would result in good, harm, or just squandered time and money.

IS THIS VALID GUIDELINE APPLICABLE TO MY PATIENT/PRACTICE/HOSPITAL/COMMUNITY?

The first (and most important) advice here is that if a guideline developed out of town tells us how to treat our patients in town, we should be very wary about its applicability. Good guideline development clearly separates the evidence component ("here's what you can expect to achieve in the typical patient who accepts this intervention") from the detailed recommendations component ("admit to an intensive care/treatment unit (ITU), carry out this ELISA test, order that Rx, monitor it minute by minute, and have your neurosurgeon examine the patient twice a day").[‡] What if we have no ITU, can't afford ELISA tests, have to fly-in the Rx, are caring for patients whose next of kin doesn't like this sort of Rx, are chronically short-staffed, and our nearest neurosurgeon is 3 hours away?

The applicability of a guideline depends on the extent to which it is in harmony or conflict with four local (sometimes patient-specific) factors, and these are summarized as the potential "killer Bs" of Table 7.4. If you hear any of these

---

[‡] Note that Cochrane Reviews recognize that they can never know the local Bs and confine themselves to summarizing the evidence compartments of the interventions they have studied.

Table 7.4 The killer Bs

1. Is the *Burden* of illness (frequency in our community, or our patient's pre-test probability or expected event rate [PEER]) too low to warrant implementation?

2. Are the *Beliefs* of individual patients or communities about the value of the interventions or their consequences incompatible with the guideline?

3. Would the opportunity cost of implementing this guideline constitute a bad *Bargain* in the use of our energy or our community's resources?

4. Are the *Barriers* (geographic, organizational, traditional, authoritarian, legal, or behavioral) so high that it is not worth trying to overcome them?

four bees buzzing in your ear when you consider the applicability of a guideline, be cautious.

First, is the *Burden* of illness too low to warrant implementation? Is the target disorder rare in our area (e.g. malaria in northern Canada)? Or is the outcome we hope to detect or prevent unlikely in our patient (e.g. the pre-test probability for significant coronary stenosis in a young woman with non-coronary chest pain)? If so, implementing the guideline may not only be a waste of time and money, but it might also do more harm than good.

Second, are our patients' or community's *Beliefs* about the values or utilities of the interventions themselves, or the benefits and harms they produce, compatible with the guideline's recommendations? The values assumed in a guideline, either explicitly or implicitly, may not match those in our patient or our community. Even if the values seem, on average, to be reasonable, we must avoid forcing them on individual patients. This is because patients with identical risks may not have the same beliefs, values and preferences as those that are used or assumed in the guideline, and some may be quite averse to undergoing the recommended procedures. For example, early breast cancer patients with identical risks, given the same information about chemotherapy, make fundamentally different treatment decisions based on how they weigh the long-term benefit of reducing the risk of recurrence against the short-term harm of being nauseated and losing their hair.[8] Similarly, severe angina patients at identical risk of coronary events, given the same information about treatment options, exhibit sharply contrasting treatment preferences because of the different values they place on the risks and benefits of surgery.[9] Although the average beliefs in a community are appropriate for deciding, for example, whether chemotherapy or surgery should be paid for with public funds, decisions for individual patients must reflect their own personal beliefs and preferences.

Third, would the opportunity cost of implementing this guideline (rather than some other one(s)) constitute a *Bargain* in the use of our energy or our community's resources? We need to remember that the cost of shortening the waiting list for surgery is lengthening that for family therapy. As decision-making of this sort gets decentralized, different communities are bound to make different economic decisions, and "health care by postal code" will and ought to occur, especially under democratic governments.

And finally, are there insurmountable *Barriers* to implementing the guideline in our patient (whose preferences generate a LHH[§] less than 1, or who would flatly refuse the investigations or intervention) or in our community? Barriers can be geographic (if the required interventions are not available locally), organizational (one of us visited a hospital with its accident and emergency rooms in the basement, its coronary care unit seven floors and 45 minutes away, and a regulation prohibiting thrombolysis in the former!), traditional ("But we've always done it the other way!"), authoritarian ("But you've always done it my way!"), legal (fear of litigation if a usual but useless practice is abandoned), or behavioral (when clinicians fail to apply the guideline or patients fail to take their medicine). If there are major barriers, the potential benefits of implementing a guideline may not be worth the effort and resources (or opportunity costs) required to overcome them.

[§] The derivation of the individual patient's LHH (Likelihood of being Helped vs. Harmed by an intervention) is described on page 124.

Changing our own, our colleagues', and our patients' behavior often requires much more than simply knowing what to do. If implementing a guideline requires changing behavior, we need to identify which barriers are operating and what we can do about them. The effects of strategies for helping both clinicians[10] and patients[11] modify their behaviors have been summarized in systematic reviews carried out within the Cochrane Collaboration, and those that apply to patients are summarized on page 131 (the bit on compliance in Ch. 5).

So, in deciding whether a valid guideline is applicable to our patient/practice/hospital/community, we need to identify the 4 Bs that pertain to the guideline and decide whether they can be reconciled with its application (or whether we are facing one or more killer Bs).

Note that none of these Bs (even when present as "killer Bs") has any effect on the validity of the evidence component of the guideline. Note also that the only people who are "experts" in the Bs are the patients and providers at the sharp edge of implementing the application component.

WHAT SHOULD I DO IF I'M ASKED TO JOIN A GUIDELINE DEVELOPMENT GROUP?

We hope, based on the foregoing, that you see how doubly dumb it is for one or a small group of local clinicians to try to create the evidence component of a guideline all by themselves. Not only are we ill-equipped and inadequately resourced for this task, but by taking it on we steal time and energy away from operationalizing our real area of expertise: knowing the local (indeed, sometimes patient-specific) burden, beliefs, bargains, and barriers that are vital to determining whether the guideline applies at all to our patient, practice, hospital, or community and, if so, how. This chapter closes with the admonition to frontline clinicians: when it comes to lending a hand with guideline development, work as a "B-keeper", not a meta-analyst.

References

1   Institute of Medicine. Clinical practice guidelines: directions for a new program. National Academy Press, Washington, DC, 1990.

2 (For example) Grimshaw J, Eccles M. Clinical practice guidelines. In: Silagy C, Haines A (eds) Evidence based practice in primary care. BMJ Publishing Group, London, 1998, pp. 110–22.

3 The Canadian Task Force on the Periodic Health Examination. The periodic health examination. Can Med Assoc J 1979; 121: 1093–254.

4 Guyatt G H, Sackett D L, Sinclair J C, Hayward R, Cook D J, Cook R J, for the Evidence-Based Medicine Working Group. Users' guides to the medical literature. IX. A method for grading health care recommendations. JAMA 1995; 274: 1800–4.

5 Ball C, Phillips R, Shenker N (eds). Evidence-based on-call. Churchill Livingstone, London, 2000.

6 Hayward R S A, Wilson M C, Tunis S R, Bass E B, Guyatt G. Users' guide to the medical literature. VII. How to use clinical guidelines. A: Are the recommendations valid? JAMA 1995; 274: 570–4.

7 Wilson M C, Hayward R S A, Tunis S R, Bass E B, Guyatt G. Users' guide to the medical literature. VII. How to use clinical guidelines. B: What are the recommendations and will they help you in caring for your patients? JAMA 1995; 274: 1630–2.

8 Levine M N, Gafni A, Markham B, MacFarlane D. A bedside decision instrument to elicit a patient's preference concerning adjuvant chemotherapy for breast cancer. Ann Intern Med 1992; 117: 53–8.

9 Nease R F, Kneeland T, O'Connor G T et al. Variation in patient utilities for outcomes of the management of chronic stable angina: implications for clinical practice guidelines. JAMA 1995; 273: 1185–90.

10 NHS Centre for Reviews and Dissemination. Getting evidence into practice. Effective Health Care 1999; 5(1): 1–16.

11 Haynes R B, Montague P, Oliver T, McKibbon K A, Brouwers M C, Kanani R. Interventions for helping patients to follow prescriptions for medications (Cochrane Review). In: The Cochrane Library, Issue 3. Update Software, Oxford, 1999.

We've already provided snippets on teaching methods when they fit the themes of previous chapters (e.g. the educational Rx in Ch. 1 and the CATs in Ch. 5) and you can find them in the index or by scanning the page margins for the mortar board icon. In this chapter, we'll present some additional strategies and tactics for teaching learners how to practice EBM. We'll begin by making explicit some of our general notions about learning and teaching, and then apply them to a number of teaching situations in which we commonly find ourselves. We'll close with a monster table of "tips" for teaching EBM (or anything else) in clinical teams and other small groups.

We're teachers of clinical medicine, not educational theorists. The educational theorists we respect and who have taken the time to understand us tell us that we don't adhere to a single dominant adult learning theory (such as behavioral, cognitive or social learning theories). Rather, we mix elements of these differing approaches and emphasize interactive and learner-centered activities for motivated, self-directed learners. Our seven general notions about teaching EBM are listed in Table 8.1 (and discussed below).

Table 8.1 Our general notions about teaching and learning EBM

Teaching and learning EBM should and can:
1. be patient-centered
2. be learner-centered
3. be active and interactive
4. be modeled as essential to becoming an expert clinician
5. match, and take advantage of, the clinical setting and circumstances
6. be well-prepared
7. be multi-staged

1. Teaching and learning EBM should be patient-centered

Practicing EBM, and therefore also learning EBM, should begin and end with patients. Over the years, our most enduring and successful teaching efforts have been those that centered on the illnesses of patients directly under the care of our learners. The clinical needs of these patients serve as the starting point for identifying our knowledge needs, and when we become adept at asking clinical questions, we can focus our learning and teaching on material that is directly relevant to these clinical needs. Further, by returning to our patients' problems after searching and appraising evidence about them, we can demonstrate how to integrate evidence with other knowledge and patient preferences.

2. Teaching and learning EBM should be learner-centered

We think teaching means helping learners learn, and we think of ourselves as learning guides and coaches, rather than dispensers of immutable truth. Since clinical learners will vary widely in their motivations, their starting knowledge, their learning styles and skills, their learning contexts and available time for learning, we need to employ a wide variety of tactics. One size does not fit all, and practitioners (and teachers!) of EBM are made, not born. We need to be patient with our learners and ourselves, allowing sufficient time for each developmental stage. To coach learners as they develop, we need to be able to "teach slow", i.e. to teach at the pace of learners' understanding. This does not mean that all learners are slow, but that we should adjust our teaching to match their pace and developmental stage. Also, we need to be willing to "teach long", i.e. to take a patient, developmental approach toward mastery. Finally, some clinical learners (especially early in their careers) have externally imposed demands they must satisfy, like cramming for exams or attending lectures. We need to acknowledge these conflicting demands, help learners cope with them, and match our tactics to their particular clinical and learning circumstances.

3. Teaching and learning EBM should be active and interactive

Learning for the "deep understanding" demanded of clinicians requires that learners actively construct their own, personal meaning of the things they learn and integrate it with their prior knowledge and skills. Clinicians, once qualified, bear the responsibility for achieving the "deep understanding" required to maintain their clinical competency. Because the ability to execute this sort of active learning must itself be learned, its principles should be introduced early in medical school. As their skills grow, learners can do more of the work of learning themselves, improving both their competence and their confidence. Interacting with peers and teachers reinforces this active process, and reinforces the learner-centered notion described above.

4. Teaching EBM should model it as essential to becoming an expert clinician

Most of our learners want to be better, faster, happier clinicians. They aspire to clinical excellence, and they respect teachers who model expert behavior and help them grow toward that goal. Teaching EBM should therefore occur implicitly through modeling, seamlessly incorporating the finding, appraisal, integration and use of evidence along with other knowledge and skill, so that learners see using evidence as a central element of, rather than separate from, routine clinical care. If we show them how powerful and useful evidence-based approaches are for carrying out their clinical work, they can more readily understand why they might be more effective clinicians if they learned the strategies and tactics of EBM (because such an approach can be so seamless as to be missed, it can be followed by debriefing, in which we make the process explicit). Moreover, this modeling reinforces learners' actual use of evidence (and its absence may negatively reinforce it). This notion does not mean that only clinicians can teach EBM skills. Non-clinicians have much to teach learners about EBM (especially around searching and advanced issues in critical appraisal), and will be more successful doing this if they emphasize the clinical uses of what they teach (pairing clinician and non-clinician teachers, especially by adding the latter to clinical teams, can lead to productive and enjoyable learning).

5. Teaching EBM should match, and take advantage of, the clinical setting and circumstances

Each patient and clinical setting defines a different learning context, where things like the severity of illness, the pace of work, the available time and person-power all combine to determine what can be learned and when, where, how and by whom it is learnt. Teaching tactics that work well in one setting (say, the outpatient clinic) may not fit at all in other settings (say, the intensive care unit). We can improve patient- and learner-centered learning by capitalizing on the opportunities that present themselves in these different settings and circumstances *as they occur*, not later. Also, especially when time is short and the patient list is long, we need to be willing to "teach small", limiting our input to just those EBM strategies that are essential to that patient.

6. Teachers of EBM should and can be well prepared

Just because EBM teaching starts and ends with today's patient, that doesn't mean that key resources and infrastructures can't be prepared in advance. First, as we showed you in Chapter 1, we can anticipate many of the questions learners will ask about the sorts of patients and clinical conditions we see commonly, so that we can gather and appraise evidence appropriate to their diagnostic tests and therapeutic interventions. By keeping CATs or other summaries of those appraisal efforts handy, we can enhance both the "teach small" and more leisurely learning. In the former situation, when the need for evidence is acute or the teaching opportunity is short, they provide the answer and model evidence-based care. In the latter situation, they can be withheld while learners fill educational prescriptions and create their own summaries and then be provided for comparison and evaluation. Second, we can create an effective learning environment for EBM by making evidence and the means to access it immediately available at the sites of care (anything less convenient than the bedside or examining room leads to a precipitous decline in its use).* Third, we can cultivate relationships with those who can help us, including librarians and clinical pharmacists, and even have them join us for rounds. Finally, we can attend one of the growing numbers of workshops on how to teach EBM (an up-to-date list can be found via this book's website: <http://www.library.utoronto.ca/medicine/ebm/>).

---

* Ideally this means fast searching computers, printers and projectors, but it can begin with a loose-leaf notebook of pertinent, up-to-date CATs.

7. Learning EBM should and can be multi-staged

As busy clinicians, we learn best what we encounter and use repeatedly. Also, rather than cram everything into a single session, we learn best when we have a chance to reflect upon, integrate and use new knowledge and skills before going on to next steps. Striving for "educational closure" by the end of a session not only cuts off problem-based learning, but also leaves the impression that learning only occurs during such sessions. Rather, when a first encounter leads us to formulate a clinical question with our learners, we can encourage the follow-through to searching, critical appraisal and application after that session closes and before the next one opens. This allows learners to try their hands at the next steps, coming to the next encounter with experiences that can be used to set its objectives.

Having described these notions, we'll now get specific by suggesting some specific strategies and tactics for teaching EBM in several common clinical teaching settings.

TEACHING AND LEARNING EBM ON THE IN-PATIENT SERVICE

There are at least seven different sorts of "rounds" that the authors have conducted (or survived) on an in-patient service, and we've summarized them in Table 8.2 (readers with additions to this list are welcome to contribute them to this book's website <http://www.library.utoronto.ca/medicine/ebm/>). Each derives a unique benefit from evidence, but each also places unique restrictions (usually time) on its incorporation into the care of patients.

We hope that Table 8.2 is self-explanatory, and will confine this text to describing the EBM strategies and resources that we use during them. Rounds on newly admitted patients ("post-take" or "admission" rounds) usually have time only for quick demonstrations of evidence-based bits of the clinical exam and how to get from pre-test to post-test probabilities of the candidate diagnosis, plus instantly available (<10 seconds) evidence about the key diagnostic and treatment decisions that have been, are being, or ought to be carried out. For example, on the Sackett–Straus service at Oxford, paper summaries carried on admission ("post-take") rounds provided

Table 8.2 Sorts of in-patient rounds

Type of round	Objectives[a]	Evidence of highest relevance	Restrictions[b]	Strategies
"Post-take" or admission rounds (after every period on call, all over the hospital, by on-call team and consultant)	Decide on working diagnosis and immediate Rx of newly admitted patients	Accuracy and precision of the clinical examination and other diagnostic tests; efficacy and safety of initial Rx	Time, motion (can't stay in one spot), and fatigue of on-call team	Demonstrate evidence-based (EB) exam and getting from pre-test to post-test probability; carry a loose-leaf book of relevant CATs; write educational prescriptions; add a clinical librarian to the team
Morning report (every day, sitting down, by entire medical service)	Briefly review new patients and discuss and debate the process of evaluating and managing one or more of them	Accuracy and precision of the clinical examination and other diagnostic tests; efficacy and safety of initial Rx	Time	Sit down in a room with a net-linked[c] computer, projector, and printer; write educational prescriptions; review old and new CATs; give 1-minute summaries on critical appraisal, NNT, etc.
Work rounds (every day, on one or several wards, by trainees)	Examine every patient and determine their current clinical state; review and (re)order tests and Rx	Accuracy and precision of diagnostic tests, efficacy and safety of ongoing Rx, and interactions	Time and motion	Create electronic links between diagnostic results or Rx orders and the relevant evidence

Table 8.2 (cont'd)

Consultant walking rounds (1–2 times a week, on one or several wards, by trainees and consultant)	As in work rounds, but objectives vary widely by consultant	As in work rounds, plus those resulting from individual consultant's objectives	Time; relevance to junior members ("shifting dullness")	Model the presentation and discussion of evidence with patients (LHH, etc)
Review "card" rounds (every day, sitting down and at the bedside, by trainees and consultant)	45-second reviews of each patient's diagnosis, Rx, progress, and discharge plans; identification of complicated patients who require bedside exam and more discussion	Wherever the educational prescriptions have led the learners	Time	Sit down in a room on the ward with a net-linked computer, projector, and printer; fill educational prescriptions; review old and new CATs; give 1-minute summaries on critical appraisal, NNT, etc.; audit whether you are following through with EB care
Social issues rounds (periodically, by trainees and a host of other professionals)	Review of each patient's status, discharge plan, referral, and post-hospital follow-up	Efficacy and safety of community services and social interventions	Time, availability of relevant participants, and necessity to meet each other's needs	Ask other health professionals to create CATs for what they routinely propose

Table 8.2 (cont'd)

Type of round	Objectives[a]	Evidence of highest relevance	Restrictions[b]	Strategies
"Pure" education rounds (1–2 times a week, by learners (often stratified) and teacher)	Develop and perfect examination and presentation skills	Accuracy and precision of the clinical examination	Time and teacher's energy and other commitments	Practice presentation and feedback; check accuracy and precision of examination skills; fill educational prescriptions; review old and new CATs; give extended summaries on critical appraisal, NNT, etc.
"Dead time" during any round	Wait for the elevator or for a report or for a team member to show up, catch up, answer a page, get off the phone, auscultate a patient, etc.	No limit	Imagination and ingenuity	Resuscitate with a recent, relevant "nugget" from an EB journal or website

[a] Increasingly, all rounds include the objective of discharging patients as soon as possible.

[b] All rounds require confidentiality when discussions of individual patients occur in public areas.

[c] The network should at least supply pre-appraised sources such as Best Evidence, The Cochrane Library, and the like.

access within seconds to one-page summaries of three-quarters of the RCT evidence we used to treat our patients.[†] When the evidence wasn't to hand, we wrote sufficient educational prescriptions to maximize the amount of appraised evidence that could reasonably be expected from our team members,[‡] and the clinical librarian on our team was invaluable in helping them master searching for the best evidence. This behavior is reinforced when modeled by the leader of the team.

In many centers, the individual teams' post-take rounds are supplemented by a service-wide, sit-down "morning report". Since not every admission has to be discussed, this round can focus on patients who have the most to teach us, and additional time can be spent confirming and increasing everyone's skills in searching and critical appraisal. When held in a permanent site, useful resources such as internet links, computer projectors and printers can be built in and always available.

"Work rounds", in which the junior staff carry out the rapid, detailed, bedside review of patients' problems and progress and the review and re-ordering of their diagnostic tests and treatments, provide perhaps the most challenging, but also the most potentially fruitful, setting for incorporating EBM into patient care. Although these rounds occur in the absence of a consultant, they provide a golden opportunity, conceptually challenging but electronically trivial, to use laboratory results or treatment orders to trigger pop-ups of evidence summaries that can be acted on immediately. For example, an elevated glucose report in a patient with a myocardial infarction could trigger a flashing evidence icon whose selection would display the CAT for the DIGAMI trial (NNT to save a life in such patients at 3.4 years by giving even short-term intensive insulin therapy = 9!). Similarly, treatment orders could trigger

---

[†] See the paper: Ellis J, Mulligan I, Rowe J, Sackett D L. Inpatient general medicine is evidence based. Lancet 1995; 346: 407–10.

[‡] On our service, every team member receives at least one educational Rx a month. Those with massive clinical responsibility (typically interns/house officers) may receive just one and reap the CATs generated by other team members who have more time (typically students and senior residents/registrars).

evidence about more efficacious or safer alternatives, interactions, drug warnings, and the like. Note that these systems do not require learners to recognize their evidence needs, but supply it in the context of patients in their care, reinforcing the importance of the evidence in making them better doctors. Initial pilot studies with radio-linked bedside or chart-rack computers are very encouraging and we will update them on this book's website: <http://www.library.utoronto.ca/medicine/ebm/>.

"Consultant walking rounds", in addition to their other important teaching functions (including especially the bedside examination), provide an excellent opportunity for the consultant to model how to combine evidence with patients' values and expectations in making management decisions. For example, this is an ideal situation in which to model applying the likelihood of being helped vs. harmed (LHH) by a treatment under consideration that we showed you in Chapter 5.

In addition to work rounds by the juniors, many consultants (some of whom keep note cards on each patient) lead brief (< 1 hour) frequent (e.g. daily, when not "on take") "review rounds" of all patients on the service. This has been most fruitful for us when we held it in a work/seminar room right on the ward. Patients are summarized in four quick phrases (what they've got, what we're doing about it, how they are doing, when and where they are going), and this quick review is interrupted for only two reasons. The first reason is when a patient is so sick or unstable or so problematic that he or she needs to be examined by the whole team every day. The second interruption is for evidence injections. These may be precipitated by any team member and are of three sorts: first, challenges (the more vigorous the better) to provide evidence that the evaluation or management decisions being made for a patient are valid and appropriate; second, quick responses (often in the form of CATs) to earlier challenges from previous rounds; and third, very brief demonstrations of the critical appraisal or application of evidence to specific patients. When the room in which these review rounds are held is equipped with a searching computer, computer projector, and printer, this presentation and sharing of evidence can be accomplished quickly and learners can go away with hard copy summaries.[§]

The "social issues rounds" provide unique opportunities for cross-professional teaching around the evidence base for the multitude of social, community and public health interventions whose impact often rivals or swamps the strictly "technical" ones.

" 'Pure' education rounds" are conducted after the patients have been cared for, and therefore enjoy the luxuries of relaxed time and choice of topic. Topics of special relevance to EBM include the more thorough bedside evaluations of the techniques, accuracy and precision of the clinical examination; more detailed learner-led discussions of how they found and appraised evidence; and the more detailed explanation and practice of skills such as generating patient-specific NNTs and NNHs. When these rounds are directed to new clinical clerks, they can include mastery of the orderly, thorough presentation of patients resident on the service, along the lines shown in Table 8.3.

Finally, all rounds of teams of size n are peppered with "dead times" that interrupt the learning process and annoy at least $(n - 1)$ of its members. Rather than permit learning to run down or be replaced by thoughts of lunch and sore backs, teachers can resuscitate these dead times by injecting nuggets of evidence from a recent evidence-based journal or website visit, perhaps accompanied by a handout. Because no learner wants to be excluded from receiving such nuggets, this tactic also encourages every team member to avoid being the cause of future dead times.

TEACHING AND LEARNING EBM IN THE OUTPATIENT CLINIC

Time both hampers and favors teaching in the outpatient setting. On the one hand, the individual outpatient appointment is short, constraining both the number and

---

[§] The provision of printouts to North American clinical teams is sometimes characterized as fulfilling the Amerindian admonition that "the photocopy is the wampum of clinical teaching".

Table 8.3 A guide for learners presenting an "old" patient at follow-up rounds

The presentation should summarize 20 things in 2 minutes:

1. The patient's name.

2. The patient's age.

3. The patient's sex.

4. The patient's occupation/social role.

5. When the patient was admitted.

6. The chief complaint(s) that led to admission.

7. The number of active problems (can be a symptom, sign, event, diagnosis, injury, psychological state, social predicament, etc.) the patient has at present.

And for each active problem:

8. Its most important symptoms, if any.

9. Its most important signs, if any.

10. The results of diagnostic or other investigations.

11. The explanation (diagnosis or state) for the problem.

12. The treatment plan instituted for the problem.

13. The response to this treatment plan.

14. The future plans for managing this problem.

[Repeat 8–14 for each active problem.]

15. Your plans for discharge, post-hospital care and follow-up.

16. Whether you've filled the educational prescription that you requested when this patient was admitted (in order to better understand the "background" of this patient's condition, or the "foreground" of how best to care for this patient with this disorder).

If so:

17. How you found the relevant evidence.

18. What you found. The clinical bottom line from that evidence.

19. Your critical appraisal of that evidence for its validity, importance and applicability.

20. How that critically appraised evidence will alter your care of that (or the next similar) patient.

If not:

17a. When you are going to fill it.

breadth of clinical and learning issues that can be addressed during any single visit. On the other hand, an outpatient's illness and its care typically comprise several visits that provide interludes for extensive learning.

The types of rounds that occur in outpatient areas are summarized in Table 8.4 and, once again, we will focus on the EBM teaching strategies and resources appropriate to each of them.

The "pre-clinic conferences", typically devoted to reviewing the diagnosis and management of common outpatient disorders, can abandon passive annual lectures on headache and chronic obstructive airways disease and (employing a system analogous to the journal club described in the next section) devote themselves to debating this year's new CATs and updating last years' old CATs (all of them created and updated by the learners themselves, perhaps with senior trainees helping their junior colleagues). Active learning occurs, and the most relevant results can be synthesized into evidence-based protocols or guidelines.

Initial outpatient visits share objectives and constraints with "post-take" rounds on new in-patient admissions, so the same strategies apply. These are quick demonstrations of evidence-based bits of the clinical exam and how to get from pre-test to post-test probabilities of the initial diagnosis, plus instantly available (<10 seconds) evidence about the key diagnostic and treatment decisions that have been, are being, or ought to be carried out.

Follow-up visits usually occur long enough after initial visits for learners to accomplish substantial problem-based learning in the interim. The lengthened episodes of care that constitute outpatient medicine provide one of the finest opportunities for multi-stage learning. When the learner first encounters an ambulatory patient, the teacher can guide the learner through the process of asking an answerable clinical question about one of this patient's problems and writing an educational Rx. At subsequent clinic sessions (and before the patient's follow-up visit), the teacher can review the learner's search strategies and critical appraisal of the evidence found. At the time of patient

Table 8.4 Sorts of outpatient rounds

Type of round	Objectives	Evidence of highest relevance	Restrictions[a]	Strategies
Pre-clinic conference (before each half-day session, by small group of learners and attendings)	Review the diagnosis and management of common outpatient disorders	Manifestations of disease, accuracy and precision diagnostic tests, efficacy and safety of therapy	Time, tardiness and duties elsewhere	Develop, debate and update CATs on the common disorders
Preceptorship during initial visits	Decide on working diagnosis and initial therapy	Accuracy and precision of clinical exam and diagnostic tests; efficacy and safety of initial Rx	Time, incomplete information	Demonstrate evident-based (EB) exam and getting from pre-test to post-test probability; provide pre-assembled CATs or other EB resources on diagnosis and initial Rx; write educational prescriptions
Preceptorship during follow-up visits	Review current status and adjust ongoing therapy	Long-term prognosis; efficacy and safety of alternative treatment options; harms from treatment	Time and changing patient needs	Model incorporation of patients' values into LHH; fill educational prescriptions

Table 8.4 (cont'd)

| Ambulatory morning report (1–3 per week), by entire outpatient service | Review the case of a particular outpatient | Anything; most common are diagnostic tests and treatment options | Time; interruptions; widely varying levels of experience | Sit down in a room with a net-linked[b] computer, projector, and printer; write educational prescriptions; review old and new CATs; give 1-minute summaries on critical appraisal, NNT, etc. |

[a] All rounds require confidentiality when discussions of individual patients occur in public areas.

[b] The network should at least supply pre-appraised sources such as Best Evidence, The Cochrane Library, and the like.

follow-up, the teacher and the learner can discuss how to integrate the evidence into clinical decisions and actions. The learner can then be asked to write a summary of the evidence in the form of a CAT (to be placed in the growing practice library of CATs), which the teacher and learner can review together at yet another clinic session. Following up on learning in this way doesn't take long at each stage, yet over time can lead to cumulative learning of EBM skills.

Finally, some teaching outpatient departments hold "morning reports" similar to those held on the inpatient service. They labor under the same restrictions, but also offer the same rich variety of opportunities for teaching and learning.

OTHER EDUCATIONAL EVENTS

Journal club

Journal clubs are dying or dead in many clinical centers, especially when they rely on a rotating schedule by which members are asked to summarize the latest issues of pre-assigned journals. Such a journal club is run by the postman, not the clinicians or patients, and it is no wonder that it is becoming extinct. On the other hand, a few journal clubs are flourishing and a growing number of them are designed and conducted along EBM lines. Each meeting of the journal club has three parts:

1. In part 1, journal club members describe patients who exemplify clinical situations which they are uncertain how best to diagnose or manage. This discussion continues until there is consensus that a particular clinical problem, which we'll call problem C, is worth the time and effort necessary to find its solution. The group may then pose one or more answerable clinical questions (usually "foreground" ones, as in Ch. 1), the answers to which should help the group build sensible approaches to the clinical problem. Group members then take responsibility (either volunteering or on rotation) for performing a search for the best evidence on problem C. Groups may have members do this in pairs or triplets, so more experienced members can teach skills to newer folks.

2. In part 2, the results of the evidence search on the previous session's problem (we'll call it problem B) are shared in the form of photocopies of the abstracts of four to six systematic reviews, original articles or other evidence. Club members decide which one or two pieces of evidence are worth studying and arrangements are made to get copies of the clinical question statement and best evidence to all members well in advance of the next meeting.

3. The main part of the journal club session (part 3) is spent in a critical appraisal of the evidence found in response to a clinical question posed two sessions ago (in response to problem A) and selected for detailed study last session. But this segment usually begins with the admission that most of the learners haven't read the articles. Rather than exclude them, everyone is given time (6 – 10 minutes) to see if they can determine the validity and clinical applicability of one of the articles (making a virtue of necessity) and reinforcing rapid critical appraisal** After that interlude, the evidence is critically appraised for its validity, importance and applicability and a decision is made about whether and how it could be applied to that or future patients by members of the journal club. This is the "pay-off" part of the session, so members have to be sure to complete parts 1 and 2 quickly in order to finish part 3. A CAT can be generated along the way (ideally drafted between sessions 2 and 3 by the member who is "it"), discussed at session 3, and then revised (if necessary) and distributed to all journal club members or posted on the group's web site.

The actual order of these three parts of the journal club meeting could be reversed, depending on local preferences and tardiness!

Group sessions ("academic half days")

Many centers bring postgraduate learners across clinical teams into regularly scheduled educational sessions. Attendance

---

** With the adoption of the "more informative abstract" by increasing numbers of journals, learners soon recognize that the answers to most of the guides for validity and importance appear in abstracts.

ranges from a handful to a hall-full, and relegating them to a series of annually recurring "canned" lectures taxes the ability of teachers to stay enthused and the willingness of learners to show up and stay awake. An alternative approach builds on the notions of teaching and learning EBM that opened this chapter and runs as follows:

1. Learners are asked to identify patients on the service whose presentations raised uncertainties about the best way to diagnose or manage them. In phrasing their uncertainties in the form of clinical questions, as in Chapter 1, learners perfect their skills in this first step of practicing EBM. Training programs employing this approach report that, early on, postgraduates identify medical emergencies in which they are unsure of their skills in diagnosing and managing life-threatening situations, and meet these concerns with early provision of advanced cardiac and/or trauma support training and sessions on the recognition and early care of patients with medical emergencies. Once this is done, attention turns to the problems of the more typical patients admitted to the service.

2. When several learners identify the same clinical problem, it joins the schedule as the topic of a future session, and the following steps (similar to those of an EBM journal club) are carried out:

   (a) Acting in rotation, one to three learners become "it" and take responsibility for searching the clinical literature for valid, relevant systematic reviews or primary articles that address the clinical question. Along the way, with help as needed from each other, from clinical faculty and from librarians, they develop and hone their skills in searching for the best evidence.

   (b) With faculty guidance, they pick the one or two articles of highest validity and relevance and these, introduced with a summary of the clinical problem and the question it prompted, are distributed to everyone well in advance of the next session.

   (c) As with the journal clubs we described in the previous section, most sessions will require a 6–10 minute interlude to permit (most of!) the learners to read the evidence. Then the learners who are "it", with faculty guidance as needed, lead the discussion of the validity, importance and applicability of the article's conclusions in answering the clinical question prompted by the patient. Toward the end of the session, CATs can be introduced and critiqued, and their "bottom lines" integrated with the relevant pathobiology and clinical skills. When consensus is reached that the session has answered an important, recurring question on the service, the edited CAT can be circulated, added to the departmental educational resources, posted on the wards, and even converted into a clinical protocol.

Grand rounds

Most hospitals hold weekly plenary sessions for all (or a departmental subset) of its members, with audiences ranging from senior consultants to clinical clerks and allied health professionals. In our view, they have deteriorated markedly in both clinical relevance and educational effectiveness over the last few decades, especially at "academic" centers: patients and demonstrations of their clinical findings have been replaced by slides showing the structure and function of molecules, membranes, and genes (highly appropriate topics for other venues but not, we suggest, as the central focus of grand rounds). When patients (usually absent) are used to introduce molecular topics, active audience participation in interrupting, challenging and debating their day-to-day clinical course, diagnostic findings and therapeutic responses frequently has been replaced by passive listening to highly censored, set-piece, uninterrupted presentations that state the final diagnosis and disposition before opening the floor to discussion. This common thread of "instructing" passive clinical audiences with facts not only ignores most clinical processes, but, as we showed you back in this book's Introduction, repeated randomized trials have shown that this approach fails to improve their subsequent clinical performance or the quality of their clinical care.

As before, reference to the educational notions that opened this chapter would combine a focus on real patients with active learning strategies shown to change clinical performance. Such grand rounds begin with the demonstration and discussion, through active audience participation, of the clinical examination of a patient at the front of the room (who may or may not stay for the rest of the round). This is followed by the similarly unvarnished and interrupted presentation of whatever other clinical data are required to set the stage for the primary discussion (e.g. diagnostic images, other diagnostic data, treatment, clinical course, or outcome). Members of the audience are asked to assess these findings, to generate opinions on their normalcy and the diagnostic, prognostic or therapeutic implications and to report their individual opinions to the assembly by shows of hands.[tt] A brief summary of the critical appraisal of the evidence that is relevant to the question posed by the round follows, again requiring the audience to offer opinions about its validity, importance and applicability. Ideally this critical appraisal is presented by a junior member of the team, demonstrating that seniority is not a prerequisite for authority. If appropriate, balloting the audience can be repeated to determine the effect of the appraisal summary on their clinical judgements. Finally, a handout[tt] is provided at the end of the round, summarizing both the relevant evidence (in the form of a CAT) and the critical appraisal guides for determining its validity, importance and applicability. For information on how to obtain a videotape of such a round conducted at the John Radcliffe Hospital in Oxford, consult the book's website: <http://www.library.utoronto.ca/medicine/ebm/>.

Lectures (for pre-clinical students and clinicians of all ages and stages)

This entry is intended for readers who are forced, by tradition, curriculum committee, or sheer numbers of learners, to use

---

[tt] The authors eliminate embarrassment and encourage participation of the junior or shy by asking members of the audience to record their opinions on blank paper or prepared forms and then exchange them with neighbors enough times that all become confident that subsequent shows of hands do *not* represent the reporters' own opinion. Some lecture halls provide anonymous keypad voting systems that speed and simplify audience participation.

[tt] Readers concerned that handouts might come across as pretentious can call them (as we do) "throw-aways".

lectures as the only or the predominant way of helping learners master the strategies and tactics of EBM. But how could lectures, especially for pre-clinical students with no clinical skills or clinical judgement, focus in an active, interactive fashion on the care of individual patients? Well, they can, based on two realizations. First, even first-year pre-clinical students already have life experiences of a wide array of illnesses: all fear contracting AIDS, most have a relative with symptomatic coronary heart disease and many know someone with breast cancer. On the first day of school, they already possess an array of personal clinical examples from which to consider the entire range of EBM topics. Second, there are teaching tactics that convert even cavernous, silent lecture halls filled with passive, somnolent students into boisterous aggregations of active learners who are surprised and delighted to discover that they are capable of making clinical decisions and supporting them with evidence.

As an example, we describe a "lecture" to 120 first-year premedical students at Oxford (videotape of this lecture can be obtained through the book's website <http://www.library.utoronto.ca/medicine/ebm/>). A real but absent "stercoraceous§§ man with a rapidly expanding belly" is presented on overheads that describe his clinical history and physical examination when first seen in the emergency room. Students are asked to form pairs and spend the next 5 minutes writing down the patient's two most important clinical findings and the two most likely explanations for his illness. During this 5-minute interval, the lecturer leaves the room for coffee. On his return (to the tumult of 60 simultaneous arguments), the students report*** their judgements and are surprised to discover their remarkable consensus on the most important findings and their likely explanation (five findings and

---

§§ Extensively soiled with, and smelling of, shit.

*** The lecturer poses the specific question – "What do you think are the two most important clinical findings I've described in this patient?" – and then *shuts up* and stares at a point at the back of the room, secure in the knowledge that within a few seconds, and with no prodding, the students will become more embarrassed than he by the awkward silence. When the response of the first pair (however off the mark) is treated positively and with respect, the floodgates open.

explanations cover >90% of their responses). Then, in open discussion, they identify the next most useful bits of diagnostic evidence, and the lecturer's reporting and interpretation of these results include an introduction (and demonstration of the clinical relevance) of precision, accuracy, pre-test probability, SpPin, SnNout, and likelihood ratios.

The diagnosis (spontaneous bacterial peritonitis, SBP[†††]), primary treatment (antibiotic), and initial response (recovery, but left with massive ascites) are discussed, and therapeutic options for the ascites nominated. Copies of a randomized trial (of repeated large-volume paracentesis vs. diuretics) are distributed and the students, in groups of four this time, are asked to take and defend a stand on whether this treatment should be offered to the patient. This time the lecturer leaves the room for a 10-minute coffee break. On return (to the roar of 30 therapeutic debates), the students report and justify their therapeutic decisions, and the ensuing discussion introduces the notion of validity and the importance of random allocation, complete follow-up, and intention-to-treat analysis (plus the observation that most of these items appeared in the article's abstract). The session is drawn to a close by observing and reinforcing self-directed problem-based learning around the clinical problems of real patients, beginning at entry to medical school. (By the way, this particular lecture was part of an introductory course in biostatistics and epidemiology – highly unpopular and subsequently redesigned. The clinical context in which the methodological concepts were raised in this session was carried over to their more detailed explanation and mastery in later sessions of this course and made them manifestly worth learning.)

TEACHING MISTAKES THAT WE HAVE MADE OR SEEN

The authors of this book have been teaching for 120 years (and have been "taught at" for close to 150). We are therefore

---

[†††] Although their explanations were unsophisticated ("some infection in his abdomen"), first-year students at Oxford suggested the correct diagnosis more often than their betters in the final year (who, when presented with the same hoof beats, ignored the pony of SBP – and failed to culture his peritoneal fluid – and pursued the zebra of "peritoneal studding with metastases from an unknown primary adenocarcinoma").

confident that we know more ways *not* to teach medicine than any of you readers. We decided that this chapter wouldn't be complete without including our top seven failures, which are listed in Table 8.5.

The first two mistakes happen when experts in any field of basic science hold (or simply fall into) the notion that in order to pragmatically apply the fruits of a science learners have to master its methods of inquiry. This is demonstrably untrue (doctors save the lives of women with breast cancer by prescribing them tamoxifen, not by learning how to perform or interpret tests for their estrogen receptors). It is also counterproductive, for it requires learners who want to become clinicians to learn the skills of transparently foreign careers, and we shouldn't be surprised by learners' indifference and hostility to courses in statistics, epidemiology and the like. Our recognition of these mistakes explains why there is so little about statistics in this book (and most of that in an appendix) and why our emphasis throughout is on how to use research reports, not how to generate them.

The third and fourth mistakes happen when we fail to begin and end all teaching sessions with the learners' patients, and when we mistake knowing facts for knowing how to find and

Table 8.5 The top seven mistakes we've made or seen in teaching EBM

1. Teaching learners how to *do* research (rather than how to *use* it).
2. Teaching learners how to *perform* statistical analyses (rather than how to *interpret* them).
3. Teaching a pre-set series of content topics (rather than have content determined by patients' problems).
4. Evaluating learners on the basis of their retention of facts (rather than their skills in obtaining, appraising, and applying "facts" to patients).
5. Insisting on sticking to the teaching schedule when the clinical service is swamped.
6. Striving for closure by the end of every session (rather than leaving plenty to think about between sessions).
7. Devaluing team members for asking "stupid" questions or providing "ridiculous" answers.

apply them. The dire consequences of these mistakes are two: first, attempts to agree on "core knowledge" in undergraduate programs defy consensus, and the consequent attempts to teach the mammoth union of their minimally overlapping objectives rather than their manageable intersect overwhelm teachers, learners and curriculum time alike; second, evaluating learners on the basis of their recall of facts subverts the educational process into teaching them how to become good examinees at the expense of teaching them how to become good doctors. Please don't misunderstand us: we are tough evaluators. Rather, the authors of this book share a preference for and commitment to frequent, rigorous evaluations of learners' requisite skills (in the clinical examination, differential diagnosis, management, procedures, use of evidence resources, communication, and the like) in caring for their patients.

The fifth and sixth mistakes happen when we behave as if learning only occurs during formal teaching sessions. This behavior is harmful in three ways. First, it takes learners away from their patients when they most need each other. Second, it cuts off problem-solving during the sessions themselves ("We're running out of time, so I want to stop this discussion and give you the right answers"). Finally, it prevents or impairs the development of the self-directed learning skills that will be essential for continuing professional development after certification.

The seventh entry is more a psychopathological state than a mistake, and is included here because it is commonplace in most medical education programs and a source of pride in some. Such treatment of juniors by their seniors is not simply wrong in human terms – it is demonstrably counterproductive. First, there is abundant evidence that this behavior discourages the very learning we claim to foster. Second, it has been well shown that positive feedback leads to increasing effort and further improvements in performance, not only among the most gifted learners but also among their less gifted peers.

Two brief additional points about evaluation (the entire next chapter is devoted to it); first, as we have already stressed above, being nice (or merely civil) to learners is not a call for relaxed standards for assessing their clinical performance. Indeed, the authors tend to demand (and receive) higher levels of performance from our learners, and hand out more "unsatisfactory" final marks, than do most of our colleagues. But criticism, even highly negative criticism, ought to be an act of purification, not hostility. Second, evaluation should go both ways: learners should, as a matter of routine, provide feedback and suggestions to their teachers on how the latter could improve their performance[‡‡‡] (surely there ought to be a mechanism for students to provide feedback to faculty about the latter's teaching effectiveness and behavior beyond portraying them with affection or contempt in the annual student pantomime?).

LEARNING MORE ABOUT HOW TO TEACH EBM

After trying out the strategies and tactics in this chapter, you may find you'd like to continue to improve your skills in teaching EBM. More reading might help, but odds are you'd benefit most from personal coaching and feedback on your skills. Mentors or other colleagues at your home institution might be helpful (simply by silently attending your rounds and giving feedback). Even so, you may find it useful to attend one of the growing number of workshops on "How to practice and teach EBM" being held at various locations around the world. These workshops provide hands-on opportunities to develop and try out your own educational resources and to gain useful feedback on your teaching methods. Detailed workshop descriptions, up-to-date schedules, and contact information can be obtained via the website that accompanies this book: <http://www.library.utoronto.ca/medicine/ebm/>.

Evaluation of learning, practicing and teaching EBM deserves its own chapter, and it follows. We close this one with Table 8.6, a grab-bag of "teaching tips" that are employed by the authors and other teachers of EBM as they strive to help their clinical teams and other small groups master the practice of evidence-based medicine.

[‡‡‡] Whether this should be done anonymously will depend on the levels of mutual respect and trust that prevail among local learners and teachers.

Table 8.6 Tips for teaching EBM in clinical teams and other small groups[a]

Help team/group members set sensible ground rules for small group learning

Small groups can succeed in learning EBM (or anything else) if group members establish effective ways of working together. Useful ground rules include the following:

1. Members take responsibility (individually and as a group) for:
   - showing up and on time
   - learning each other's names, interests and objectives
   - respecting each other
   - contributing to, accepting and supporting individual and group rules of behavior, including confidentiality
   - contributing to, accepting and supporting both the overall objectives of the group and the detailed plans and assignments for each session
   - carrying out the agreed plans and assignments, including role-playing
   - listening (concentrating and analyzing), rather than simply preparing your own response to what's being said)
   - talking (including consolidating and summarizing).

2. Members monitor and (by using time in/time out) reinforce positive and correct negative elements of both:
   (a) "Process", including:
      - educational methods, e.g. reinforcing positive contributions and teaching methods; proposing strategies for improving less effective ones
      - group functioning, e.g. identifying behaviors, not motives; encouraging non-participants; quieting down over-participators.
   (b) "Content", including:
      - critical appraisal topics, e.g. if unclear, uncertain or incorrect facts or principles, strategies or tactics about how to carry it out
      - clinical matters, e.g. if clinical context or usefulness is unclear.

3. Members evaluate self, each other, the group, the session, and the program with candor and respect:
   - celebrating what went well and should be preserved
   - identifying what went less well, focusing on strategies for correcting or improving the situation.

4. When giving feedback constructively, members do the following:
   - Give feedback only when asked to do so or when the offer is accepted.
   - Give feedback as soon after the event as possible.
   - Focus on the positive; wherever possible give positive feedback first and last.

Table 8.6 *(cont'd)*

- Be descriptive (of behavior), not evaluative (of motives).
- Talk about specific behaviors and give examples where possible.
- Use "I" and give your experience of the behavior.
- When giving negative feedback, suggest alternative behaviors.
- Confine negative feedback to behaviors that can be changed.
- Ask, "Why am I giving this feedback?" (Is it really to help the person concerned?)
- Remember that feedback says a lot about its giver as well as its receiver.

5. When receiving feedback constructively, members do the following:

- Listen to it (rather than prepare a response or defense).
- Ask for it to be repeated if it wasn't easily heard.
- Ask for clarification and examples if statements are unclear or unsupported.
- Assume it is constructive until proven otherwise; then, use and consider those elements that are constructive.
- Pause and think before responding.
- Accept it positively (for consideration) rather than dismissively (for self-protection).
- Ask for suggestions of specific ways to modify or change the behavior.
- Respect and thank the person giving feedback.

Help team/group members plan the learning activities wisely

During initial introductions, group members should identify their individual learning goals, from which the group can set group learning goals. Tutors and group members should keep these learning goals in mind as they plan the learning objectives for each session, including what to learn, what to emphasize and how to engage the group in the learning activities. For groups just beginning to learn EBM, consider the following:

1. Plan the session to include a learning situation that is realistic to what group members do in their actual work. For most clinicians, this means using the illnesses of patients actually in their care, or case examples they might encounter frequently.

2. Prepare the question, search and critical appraisal ahead of time, to be familiar with the teaching challenges that may arise. Of the possible questions this case could generate, select one with a high yield in terms of learning, which is usually a mix of the following considerations:

- relevance to the clinical decision being made
- appropriateness to the learners' prior knowledge
- availability of good-quality evidence to address the question (so first experience shows positively how evidence can be used once understood and appraised)

Table 8.6 *(cont'd)*

- availability of easily understood evidence about the question (so first experience is not too overwhelming methodologically)
- likelihood the question will recur, so learners can benefit more than once.

3. As the session begins, engage the group in the clinical situation and have the group focus on the decision to be made. Consider having group members vote on what they would do clinically before the evidence is appraised (if need be, this can be done anonymously).

4. Encourage group members to run the session, yet be prepared to guide them in the early going.

5. As the group works through the critical appraisal portions, emphasize how to understand and use research, rather than how to do research.

6. Summarize important points in the session (if the group is using a scribe, this person could record them for later retrieval).

7. As the session ends, encourage the group to come to closure on how to use the evidence in the clinical decision. Keep in mind that coming to closure needn't require complete agreement; rather, a good airing of the issues that ends in legitimate disagreement can be very instructive.

8. Keep to the time plan overall, but don't worry if the group doesn't cover everything in this one session – if the initial experience goes well, there will be more opportunities.

9. For groups gaining competence and confidence in EBM, the sky is the limit. Encourage the group to invent its own activities, and consider the following.

   (a) When selecting questions and evidence to appraise, consider using:

   - flawed evidence, so the group can develop skill in detecting flaws
   - a pair of articles, one good and one not so good, for the group to compare
   - a pair of good articles that reach opposite conclusions
   - controversial evidence, so the group learns to disagree constructively
   - evidence that debunks current practice, so the group learns to question carefully
   - a systematic review of early small trials, along with a later definitive trial.

   (b) When selecting learning contexts to employ in the group, encourage group members to try out sessions of increasing difficulty, such as practicing teaching jaded senior residents rather than eager students.

   (c) When group members disagree, capitalize on the disagreement, by such tactics as:

Table 8.6 *(cont'd)*

- trying to sort out whether the disagreement is about the data, the critical appraisal or the values we use in making the judgements
- framing the disagreement positively, as a chance to understand more deeply
- framing the protagonists positively, as providing the group a chance to learn by stating the various perspectives on the topic
- wherever possible, keeping the disagreement from becoming personal.

Help team/group members keep a healthy learning climate

The learning climate is the general tone and atmosphere that pervades the group sessions. Encourage the group to cultivate a safe, positive learning climate, wherein group members feel comfortable identifying their limitations and addressing them. Some tactics include the following:

1. Be honest and open about your own limitations and the things you don't know.
2. Model the behavior of turning what you don't know into answerable questions and following through on finding answers, using an educational prescription.
3. Have fun with, and show others the fun in, finding knowledge gaps and learning.
4. Encourage all questions, particularly those that aim for deep understanding.
5. Encourage legitimate disagreement, particularly when handled constructively.
6. Encourage group members to use educational prescriptions.
7. Provide both intellectual challenge (to help stimulate learning) and personal support (to help make learning adaptive).

Help team/group members keep the discussion going

1. Early on, model effective facilitating behaviors that encourage discussion, such as:
   - When someone asks a question, turn the question over to the group and ask them.
   - If a group member answers another member's question well, ask others in the group for additional effective ways that they've used to answer the same question.
   - If a group discussion turns into a debate between two members, ask others to provide additional perspective before the group decides.
   - Don't be afraid of quiet moments, and of using silence when needed.

Table 8.6 (cont'd)

2. Observe carefully how group members keep discussion moving, and use these observations for feedback and coaching.

3. Encourage group members to reflect on what works well in different teaching situations, balancing the desire to move forward with the need to pull everyone along.

Help group members keep the discussion on track

1. Early on, model effective facilitating behaviors that help group members to stay focused on the task at hand, such as:

   - Break the discussion into observable chunks, and set a short time for each chunk, e.g. "For the next 2 minutes, let's brainstorm all the outcomes of clinical interest to us for this condition and its treatment."
   - When someone brings up a tangent, identify it non-judgmentally and ask the group how they'd like to handle it.
   - Reflect to the group what they seem to be discussing, to inform their choices about how to spend their efforts.

2. Observe carefully how group members keep the discussion on track, and use these observations for feedback and coaching.

3. Encourage group members to reflect on what works well for keeping a discussion focused well, while at the same time staying alert for good teaching moments that arise spontaneously.

Help team/group members manage time well

To accomplish their group objectives, group members need to manage their time together effectively. This includes spending time on things that are important and avoiding distractions wherever possible. Some tactics include:

1. At the beginning, model effective time management by encouraging the group to set specific plans for how much time to spend on:

   - carrying out the learning activities for the present session
   - evaluating the present session, including giving feedback
   - planning the subsequent sessions, including revising group objectives.

2. As the group takes charge, coach the members on issues of time management, such as:

   - how to use a "timekeeper", usually a member not leading that session
   - how to adjust time allotted for various functions, after group negotiation
   - how to handle new learning issues that arise, which might consume time to address. Here, several options exist, including the following:

     (a) address it fully right then (if it's important enough and if the group's work would halt without doing so)

Table 8.6 *(cont'd)*

  (b) address it briefly at the time, and have a group member (or tutor) address it more completely later, either to the group or with the individual

  (c) delay addressing the topic; instead, record it for later discussion (in a place sometimes dubbed "the parking lot").

3. Encourage the group to evaluate time management as the members evaluate the group's functioning.

Help team/group members address some common issues of learning EBM

Jargon

Jargon consists of words from the technical languages of any discipline; for EBM these can be from epidemiology, biostatistics, decision sciences, economics and other fields. If unexplained, jargon can be intimidating and might delay learning. Some tactics for dealing with jargon include:

1. Introduce and explain the idea first, then label it with the technical term. In this way the understanding comes first, before the word can intimidate.

2. If group members introduce jargon terms, ask them to explain the terms to the others in concise ways. This helps the group's understanding, and allows the member to practice brief explanations for later use.

3. Consider having the group keep an accumulating glossary of terms covered, for members to refer to during and after the sessions. You can start with the brief glossary that is in each issue of evidence-based journals such as *ACP Journal Club* and databases such as Best Evidence.

Quantitative study results

Most reports contain simple calculations, and many contain complex and intimidating ones. Although most of them don't deserve extensive discussion, others, if left unexplained, can needlessly intimidate some learners. Tactics for dealing with quantitative results include:

1. Introduce the concept using real data and working slowly through the arithmetic, so learners can follow the calculations.

2. Use the word names for the arithmetical functions, rather than talking in symbols.

3. Calculate a result from the study data, and then introduce its name and a general formula. Just as in dealing with jargon, this order helps to demystify the terms.

4. To check their understanding, allow group members time to practice the arithmetic until they feel comfortable enough to move on.

5. Consider having the group keep an accumulating glossary of quantitative results, including names, formulae and uses, for group members to use during and afterwards. Again, the glossaries of EB journals can provide the nidus for this activity.

Table 8.6 *(cont'd)*

Statistics

The study's methods and results sections will usually describe the technical devices of statistics used for the research. Some may be familiar to you and your group members, while many may not be. Groups will need to learn how to handle questions about statistics, epidemiology, or any other methodological issue; some tactics include:

1. Highlight the distinction between statistical and clinical significance, and illustrate with evidence being examined.

2. Assuming the group members want to learn how to understand and use research, rather than do research (worth double-checking now and then), consider advising the group to select a few statistical notions to understand well (e.g. confidence intervals), and point them to resources that can help them (such as the appendix on confidence intervals in this book).

3. Ask the group how deeply they'd like to delve into this topic (many will opt for shallow initial treatment, to allow the group's work to continue, followed by resources for deeper learning later). If they choose deeper amounts, and you cannot provide this on the spot, involve them in choosing among the realistic alternatives, including:

   • A single group member (or the tutor, if needed) looks up the statistical measure or test and reports back concisely at a later session.

   • Pairs or small teams from the group find the needed information outside of the session, and plan a learning activity around it for a subsequent session,

   • A nearby statistician is persuaded to join the group temporarily to address the topic at a subsequent session.

4. Remind group members that they may face learners with similar questions upon return home. Coach them in developing answers of different lengths and depths, appropriate for different situations:

   • "one-liners" – for when learners want just enough to get back to other work

   • "one-paragraphers" – for when learners want more verbal explanation

   • "one-siders" – one-page (or a few) handouts on the topic that might be developed ahead of time, for learners who want a little more depth to read later; this can be coupled with "one-citers", i.e. a useful citation for even more depth.

5. As the group members run sessions themselves, observe carefully how they handle statistical, epidemiological or other methodological issues and use these observations in coaching and feedback.

6. Ask the group to assess its handling of methodological topics when they evaluate it.

7. Consider having the group keep a cumulative list of methodological issues covered.

Table 8.6 *(cont'd)*

Help team/group members identify and deal with counterproductive behaviors

Nihilism

As learners grow in their ability to detect study flaws, some may go through a period of nihilism ("No study is perfect, so what good is any literature?"). Often this occurs in those who can find bias but who don't yet understand its consequences. This negative imbalance is usually temporary, but it can dampen the spirits of others and impede group function. Some tactics are useful in ameliorating this unease:

1. Select good articles at the start, so that early experiences are positive.

2. When using flawed articles, ask the group if something can be learned, even if the study doesn't provide a definitive answer.

3. Help group members put the study in its knowledge context – what else is known about this? Although potentially flawed, a study may be the earliest in a given field, when the state of prior knowledge is low. Thus, the study may represent incomplete knowledge, rather than bad knowledge.

4. Help group members ask whether missing information is due to poor study design and execution or due to editorial decisions about publishing space. Some data missing in the report may be available from the authors of the study.

5. Help group members separate minor problems from major design flaws that seriously affect the likely validity of results.

6. Help group members ask a series of questions:

   - Do the study methods allow the possibility of bias?
   - If so, how much distortion of the results might this bias cause?
   - If so, in which direction might this bias distort the results?

7. Help group members identify what they would find in an ideal study that answers the question. Then consider how far from ideal is the available evidence.

Discussion tangents

Small group work can stimulate learners, bringing forth not only discussion ideas that would keep the group on their learning spiral, but also discussion ideas that could take the group elsewhere (tangents from the spiral). The energy released can be invigorating, yet if every topic were to be discussed, the group may not achieve its objectives. Group members need to learn constructive ways of handling possible discussion tangents, some of which are as follows:

1. Identify to the group that a tangent has arisen, validating it as a possibly productive line of learning.

2. Ask the group to choose how to proceed, based on their overall learning goals rather than just the plan for that session. This may mean following the tangent, as it might meet their goals better, or it may mean placing the tangent on a list of topics to address later

Table 8.6 (cont'd)

(the "parking lot"). Either way, encourage the group to decide, letting them know you'll stick with them on either path.

3. Some tangents can be turned into extended loops of the learning spiral. That is, these topics can be briefly and concisely discussed, enough to inform the original discussion, to which the group then returns. It may help to set a time limit for such a tangent, and have the timekeeper help the group keep to the limit.

4. When they're running the session, observe closely how group members deal with tangents and use these observations for feedback and coaching.

5. Encourage the group to assess its management of tangents during its evaluation.

A dominating, over-participator

Some groups may have one or more members whose personality or enthusiasm leads them to contribute a great deal, perhaps to the point of dominating the time and impeding the group's work and the other members' learning. Some tactics for dealing with this include:

1. Use non-verbal signals (eye contact, hand gestures, body position, etc.) to encourage this person to become quieter and others to contribute more.

2. Seat this person next to one of the tutors, which can encourage moderation.

3. After this person contributes again, ask several others to contribute. This may take reminding the over-participator to let others have a fair turn to speak.

4. Take a time-out to address the group's process, perhaps by reviewing the group's ground rules about participation, or by asking the group to identify the over-participation and make adjustments. In doing so, focus on the behavior (amount and nature of speech), rather than on the person or the motivations for the behavior.

5. Consider suggesting the device of a "peace pipe". This can be any object (originally an actual tobacco pipe used at Native American gatherings) that signifies that the person holding it has permission to speak. When finished speaking, that person may give the object to someone else or place it on the table for anyone to choose. This can be a fun and instructive exercise to try, through which group members can discover both under- and over-participation, as well as how many of them talk at once.

A quiet, non-participator

Some group members are quiet initially, as they "warm up" to the people and the group's activities. Other members may be quiet longer, either from personal style or for other reasons like language skills. Still others may be quiet due to lack of preparation, for fear of embarrassment or due to lack of engagement. While not always pathologic, quietness can be a signal to individual or group troubles.

Table 8.6 (cont'd)

Groups will need tactics to recognize and address members that contribute little, some of which are:

1. Be sensitive to the reasons for quietness and adjust accordingly. If need be, approach the group member between sessions to find out why.

2. Use non-verbal signals (eye contact, hand gestures, body position, etc.) to encourage this person to contribute more.

3. Seat this person next to one of the tutors, which can encourage participation.

4. Take a time-out to address the group's process, perhaps by reviewing the group's ground rules about participation, or by asking the group to identify the under-participation and make adjustments. In doing so, focus on the behavior (amount and nature of speech), rather than on the person or the motivations for the behavior.

5. Consider pairing the quiet person with another group member for an activity, so they can work together on planning and carrying out this activity. Make sure quiet folks (and all group members) feel more supported as they take on challenges in the group.

6. Consider trying a "peace pipe" (see above). For under-participators, tutors and group members can make a point to pass it to them, asking them to contribute at least a little before passing it on to others.

Help team/group members prepare for using EBM skills "back home"

As they grow in competence and confidence in their EBM skills, group members will begin to confront how to start or advance their use of EBM in their daily work. For clinicians and teachers, this may mean facing for the first time some of the barriers to incorporating evidence in practice addressed elsewhere in this book. You can help them prepare to overcome these barriers with a mix of enthusiasm, realism and practicality. Some tactics include:

1. Encourage each group member to select one or a few places to start introducing EBM, rather than trying to start everywhere at once. Consider having them rank three or more candidate activities for introducing EBM, then discussing in buzz groups the advantages and disadvantages of each.

2. Use the group members' collective experience to brainstorm how to prepare to introduce EBM into a given learning activity. This brainstorming might be usefully organized around:

   • persons (faculty, learners, librarians, departmental leaders, etc.),

   • places (conference rooms, rounding facilities, etc.)

   • things (access to literature and critical appraisal tools, other resources, etc.),

   • times (for planning and preparation of the sessions, the sessions themselves, the debriefing and troubleshooting, etc.), that would need to be considered when introducing EBM "back home".

Table 8.6 *(cont'd)*

3. Since changes involving only a few may be easier than changes involving many, it may be wise to work toward an early success by introducing EBM in a way that doesn't require massive shifts in institutional culture. Indeed, the simplest may be a change that involves the actions of only the group member, at least at first. Once momentum is gained, more challenging tasks can be tackled.

4. Encourage group members to be realistic in setting expectations for what can be accomplished early, yet optimistic about what can be achieved in the long term.

[a] Credit for the original compilation of an earlier version of this list goes to Martha Gerrity and Valerie Lawrence, and we hope they don't mind our tinkering with it.

Further reading

1 Davis D, Thomson M A. Continuing medical education as a means of lifelong learning. In: Silagy C, Haines A (eds). Evidence-based practice in primary care, ch. 11. BMJ Books, London (UK), 1998, pp. 129–43.

2 Jason H, Westberg J. Fostering learning in small groups: a practical guide. Springer, Philadelphia, 1996.

3 Maudsley G. Roles and responsibilities of the problem based learning tutor in the undergraduate medical curriculum. Br Med J 1999; 318: 657–61.

4 Neighbour R. The inner apprentice. Petroc Press, Newbury (UK), 1996.

Evaluation

The fifth step in practicing EBM is self-evaluation and we'll suggest some approaches for doing that in this final chapter. We'll also summarize the results of external evaluations of EBM and of the different ways of teaching and learning how to practice it.

SELF-EVALUATION

As you might have guessed by now, we believe that the most important evaluations of our performance are the ones we design and carry out ourselves. Accordingly, this part of the chapter will describe the domains in which you might want to evaluate your performance. We also will note some aids to self-evaluation that you can find from the book's website.

Evaluating our performance in asking answerable questions

We'd suggest asking ourselves 10 questions, in two batches of five each (Table 9.1). The first five questions in the table are about our own question-asking in practicing EBM. First, are we asking any questions at all? As we begin to do so, are they well formulated? As our experience grows, are we using a map of where most questions come from (Table 1.2 is our version) to locate our knowledge gaps, and help us articulate questions? When we get stuck, are we increasingly able to get "unstuck" using the map or other devices? On a practical level, have we devised a method to note our questions as they occur, for later retrieval and answering when time permits?

The second five questions in Table 9.1 concern how we are doing incorporating questions into our clinical teaching. First, are we modeling for our learners how to find and acknowledge information needs and ask answerable clinical questions? Next, are we using educational prescriptions, and if so, are they being "filled" by our learners? Have we incorporated asking

9

Table 9.1 Self-evaluation in asking answerable questions

1. Am I asking any clinical questions at all?
2. Am I asking well-formulated questions:
   (a) two-part questions about "background" knowledge?
   (b) four- (or three) part questions about "foreground" diagnosis, management, etc.?
3. Am I using a "map" to locate my knowledge gaps and articulate questions?
4. Can I get myself "unstuck" when asking questions?
5. Do I have a working method to save my questions for later answering?
6. Am I modeling the asking of answerable questions for my learners?
7. Am I writing any educational prescriptions in my teaching? Are they being "filled"?
8. Are we incorporating question asking and answering into everyday activities?
9. How well am I guiding my learners in their question asking?
10. Are my learners writing educational prescriptions for me?

and answering questions into our everyday clinical work? As our learners grow in skill and confidence, how are we coaching and guiding them in asking questions? Have they reached the point where they can write educational prescriptions for us?

As we grow in asking questions and in teaching questions, we may also find some need to have the benefit of others' evaluations of our performance. We can turn to our respected colleagues and mentors for this, inviting them to observe one of our teaching sessions and discuss it with us afterward, giving us and them a chance to learn together. We might also seek out a workshop on EBM to refine our skills further (upcoming workshops can be found via this book's website: <http://www.library.utoronto.ca/medicine/ebm/>).

Evaluating our performance in searching

Table 9.2 lists some questions we might want to ask ourselves about our performance in searching for the best external evidence. Again, are we searching at all? Do we know the best sources of current evidence for our clinical discipline? Have

Table 9.2 A self-evaluation in finding the best external evidence

1. Am I searching at all?
2. Do I know the best sources of current evidence for my clinical discipline?
3. Have I achieved immediate access to searching hardware, software and the best evidence for my clinical discipline?
4. Am I finding useful external evidence from a widening array of sources?
5. Am I becoming more efficient in my searching?
6. Am I using MeSH headings, thesaurus, limiters, and intelligent free text when searching MEDLINE?
7. How do my searches compare with those of research librarians or other respected colleagues who have a passion for providing best current patient care?

we achieved immediate access to searching hardware, software and the best evidence for our clinical discipline? Will our practice or hospital or other institution put the appropriate hardware, software and resources right in the places where we do our clinical work, or is it time to bite the bullet and purchase these ourselves? If we have started searching on our own, are we finding useful external evidence from a widening array of sources, and are we becoming more efficient in our searching? For example, the authors are pretty used to firing up their laptops and hopping quickly back and forth between searches in CD-based compendia of back issues of evidence-based journals,* collections of systematic reviews (on the Cochrane Library), medical textbooks, primary publications (using one of the MEDLINE systems), national drug formularies, and the like, and have met full-time front-line clinicians who can search circles around us!

Are we using MeSH headings, thesaurus, limiters, and intelligent free text when searching MEDLINE? An efficient way of evaluating our searching skills is to ask research librarians or other respected colleagues to repeat a search that we've already done and then compare notes on both the

---

* The one two of us edit is *Best Evidence*. <http://www.bmjpg.com/data/ebm.htm>.

searching strategy and the usefulness of the evidence we both found. Done this way, we benefit in three ways: from the evaluation itself, from the opportunity to learn how to do it better, and from the yield of additional external evidence on the clinical question that prompted our search.

If we are still having problems with the efficiency and effectiveness of our searching, it would be wise to consult our nearest health sciences library about taking a course or personal tutorial, so that we can get to the level of expertise we need to carry out this second step in practicing EBM. We might even persuade one of the librarians to join our clinical team, an extraordinary way to increase our proficiency!

Evaluating our performance in critical appraisal

Table 9.3 lists some questions we can incorporate into our self-evaluation of how we are doing in critically appraising external evidence for its validity and potential usefulness. Beginning at the beginning, are we critically appraising external evidence at all? If not, can we identify the barriers to our performance and remove them? Once again, we might find that working as a member of a group (such as the different sort of journal club we describe in Ch. 8) could not only help us get going but also give us feedback about our performance.

Once we're underway, we could ask ourselves whether the critical appraisal guides are becoming easier to apply. Most clinicians find that this is the case for most of them, but identify one or two that continue to confuse. Again, this is a situation in which working in a group can quickly identify and

Table 9.3 A self-evaluation in critically appraising the evidence for its validity and potential usefulness

1. Am I critically appraising external evidence at all?

2. Are the critical appraisal guides becoming easier for me to apply?

3. Am I becoming more accurate and efficient in applying some of the critical appraisal measures (such as likelihood ratios, NNTs and the like)?

4. Am I creating any CATs?

resolve such confusion. We can then proceed to consider whether we are becoming more accurate and efficient in applying some of the critical appraisal measures (such as likelihood ratios, NNTs and the like). This could be done by comparing our results with those of colleagues who are appraising the same evidence, or by taking the raw data from an article abstracted in one of the journals of secondary publication, making the calculations, and then comparing them with the abstract's conclusions.

At the most advanced level, are we creating any CATs these days? If we use one of the "CAT-makers", how do our raw calculations compare with those that the software generates? Finally, if can we find a duplicate of the CAT we've just generated in one of the CAT libraries or databanks, we can make contacts and compare notes with a colleague who may be continents away.

Evaluating our performance in integrating evidence and patients' values

Table 9.4 lists some elements of a self-evaluation of our skills in integrating our critical appraisals with our clinical expertise and applying the results in our clinical practice. Not surprisingly, it opens by suggesting that we ask ourselves whether we are integrating our critical appraisals into our practice at all. Because the efforts we've expended in the previous three steps are largely wasted if we can't execute this

Table 9.4 A self-evaluation in integrating the critical appraisal with clinical expertise and applying the result in clinical practice

1. Am I integrating my critical appraisals into my practice at all?
2. Am I becoming more accurate and efficient in adjusting some of the critical appraisal measures to fit my individual patients (pre-test probabilities, NNT/f, etc.)?
3. Can I explain (and resolve) disagreements about management decisions in terms of this integration?
4. Have I conducted any clinical decision analyses?
5. Have I carried out any audits of my diagnostic, therapeutic, or other EBM performance?

fourth one, we'd need to do some soul-searching and carry out some major adjustments of how we spend our time and energy if we're not following through on it. Once again, talking with a mentor or working as a member of a group might help overcome this failure, as might attending one of the EBM workshops. Once we are on track, we could ask ourselves whether we are becoming more accurate and efficient in adjusting some of the critical appraisal measures to fit our individual patients. Have we been able to find or otherwise establish pre-test probabilities that are appropriate to our patients and the disorders we commonly seek in them? Are we becoming more adept at modifying measures like the NNT to take into account the "f" for our patient?

One way to test our growing skills in this integration is to see whether we can use them to explain (and maybe even resolve!) disagreements about management decisions. For example, a senior colleague of one of us recently took exception to our decision to treat a patient at low risk of embolism from her non-valvular atrial fibrillation with aspirin rather than warfarin. We were able to produce light as well as heat from the subsequent discussion by showing how different weights placed on this patient's NNT and NNH by the two of us (and by the patient!) could explain the disagreement (if not resolve it!).

Although a self-evaluation showing success at the foregoing level should bring enormous satisfaction and pride to any clinician, we might want to proceed even further, and could ask ourselves whether we have conducted any clinical decision analyses or carried out any audits of our diagnostic, therapeutic, or other EBM performance? Audits of clinical practice can be important for two reasons. First, they can tell us how we are performing as clinicians. Second, and far more important, they often incorporate strategies, especially individualized feedback, that can have a very positive effect on our clinical performance.

Audits can occur at various levels of complexity, and many hospitals have well-developed audit committees with full-time staff. Because this book is directed to individual clinicians, we won't devote space to audits carried out at these higher levels of organization.[†] Rather, we'll focus on audits that can be accomplished by individual clinicians and their teams. Given the thrust of this book, it will come as no surprise to readers to learn that we would precede any audit with a proper critical appraisal of the evidence that any clinical acts we contemplate auditing have actually been shown to result in more good than harm (or equal good for fewer resources).

Once we have valid external evidence that certain patients with certain disorders, if diagnosed and managed in certain ways, enjoy importantly improved outcomes, we have the basis for carrying out audits of that care. If, for example, we find solid evidence that patients heparinized for deep vein thrombosis fare better when they achieve therapeutic PTT levels within 24 hours of initiating therapy, we have the basis for a continuous audit of such patients when they come onto our service. Similarly, we can monitor the "door-to-needle" time for thrombolytic therapy in patients with suspected myocardial infarction, or the proportion of patients with high-risk non-valvular atrial fibrillation who are adequately anticoagulated. In addition, since patients require accurate diagnosis before they can benefit from efficacious treatment, audits of the diagnostic process are also highly appropriate activities.

But we can also carry out individual practice or team audits of the extent to which we are practicing evidence-based diagnosis or management, and as this book went to press, a number of clinical teams were doing so. The impetus for their work was the "conventional wisdom" that only about 20% of clinical care was based in solid scientific evidence.[‡] One of the first studies was performed on DLS's clinical service in Oxford, where at the time of their discharge, death, or retention in hospital at the end of the audited month, every patient was discussed at a team meeting and consensus reached on their primary diagnosis (the disease, syndrome, or condition entirely or, in the case of multiple diagnoses, most responsible

---

[†] These are described in detail in a companion text by Muir Gray (*Evidence-Based Healthcare*. Churchill Livingstone, London, 1997).

[‡] In 1963, the estimate was 9.3%! (Medical Care 1963; 1: 10–16).

for the patient's admission to hospital) and their primary intervention (the treatment or other maneuver that represented our most important attempt to cure, alleviate, or care for the primary diagnosis). The primary intervention was then traced, either into an "instant resource book of evidence-based medicine" maintained by the consultant or to other sources (medical texts, or, via computerized bibliographic database searching, into the published literature), and classified into one of three categories: interventions whose value (or non-value) is established in one or more randomized controlled trials or, better yet, systematic reviews of RCTs; interventions whose face-validity is so great that randomized trials into their value were unanimously judged by the team to be both unnecessary and, if they involved placebo treatments, unethical; and interventions in common use but failing to meet either of the preceding two criteria.

Of the 109 patients diagnosed that month, 90 (82%) were judged by pre-set criteria to have received evidence-based interventions. The primary interventions for 53% of patients were based on one or more randomized trials or systematic reviews of trials, and of the 28 randomized trials or overviews we consulted, 21 had already been summarized as CATs that were carried on post-take rounds (the other seven were identified a few hours later through literature-searching by a team member, and therefore only confirmed a previous decision). An additional 29% of patients received interventions unanimously judged to be based on convincing non-experimental evidence, and 18% received specific symptomatic and supportive care without substantial evidence that it was superior to some other intervention or to no intervention at all.

This audit both confirmed that in-patient general medicine could be evidence-based and illustrated how an established pattern of evidence-based reading around one's patients, coupled with a method for storing the fruits of that reading, could provide useful evidence at the times and places where it could be the most useful and educational.

Similar audits were carried out shortly thereafter in psychiatry, adult and pediatric surgery, pediatrics and general practice, with similar results (they are being collated and updated by Andrew Booth on his website: <http://www.shef.ac.uk/~scharr/ir/percent.html>. The truth is that most patients we encounter have one of just a few common problems, while the rare problems are thinly spread between many patients. As a result, searching for the evidence that underpins the common problems provides a greater and more useful reward for our effort than fruitless quests for evidence about problems we might encounter once a decade. That these studies have found evidence for most common interventions has validated the feasibility of the practicing EBM. The key point for readers of this book is to recognize how such audits not only focus on clinical issues that are central to providing high-quality evidence-based care but also provide a natural focus for day-to-day education, helping every member of the team keep up to date.

Evaluating our performance as teachers

Table 9.5 lists some ways of evaluating how we're doing as teachers of EBM. When did we last issue an educational prescription (or have one issued to us)? If not, why not? Are we helping our trainees learn how to ask answerable (four-part) questions? Are we teaching and modeling searching skills? Our time may be far too limited to provide this training ourselves, but we should be able to find some help for our

Table 9.5 A self-evaluation in teaching EBM

1. When did I last issue an educational prescription?
2. Am I helping my trainees learn how to ask answerable (four-part) questions?
3. Am I teaching and modeling searching skills (or making sure that my trainees learn them)?
4. Am I teaching and modeling critical appraisal skills?
5. Am I teaching and modeling the generation of CATs?
6. Am I teaching and modeling the integration of best evidence with my clinical expertise and my patients' preferences?
7. Am I developing new ways of evaluating the effectiveness of my teaching?
8. Am I developing new EBM educational material?

learners. Are we teaching and modeling critical appraisal skills, and teaching and modeling the generation of CATs? If this is proving a problem for you, maybe the software we've developed can help. Are we teaching and modeling the integration of best evidence with our clinical expertise and our patients' preferences? Are we developing new ways of evaluating the effectiveness of our teaching? Particularly important here are the development and use of strategies for obtaining feedback from our students and trainees about our skills and performance in practicing and modeling EBM. A formal system for obtaining this feedback has been in place at McMaster University in Canada (and, no doubt, elsewhere) for some time, and if you have developed useful strategies for accomplishing this, please share them with the rest of us via the book's website: <http://www.library.utoronto.ca/medicine/ebm/>! Finally, are we developing new EBM educational materials?

Evaluating our performance in our own continuing professional development

Table 9.6 suggests some ways for us to evaluate our own continuing professional development. First, are we a member of an EBM-style journal club? That's a superb way to continue to develop our skills at every step of practicing EBM. Have we participated in or tutored at one of the workshops on how to practice or teach EBM? The opportunities they provide for learning, for linking with other clinicians with similar interests, for generating educational materials, and for just plain thinking about and debating EBM are unparalleled. Have you joined the evidence-based-health e-mail discussion group?[§] As this

Table 9.6 A self-evaluation of continuing professional development

1. Am I a member of an EBM-style journal club?
2. Have I participated in or tutored at one of the workshops on how to practice or teach EBM?
3. Have I joined the evidence-based health e-mail discussion group?
4. Have I established links with other practitioners or teachers of EBM?

[§] See the book's website for instructions on how to join: <http://www.library.utoronto.ca/medicine/ebm/>.

edition was being written, this group was extremely active, exchanging sources of good evidence on pre-test probabilities, announcing all sorts of educational and job opportunities, and providing many of the ideas and examples that appear in this book.

EVALUATIONS OF STRATEGIES FOR TEACHING THE STEPS OF EBM

Having read this far, you have already encountered (in the Introduction) the outcomes research showing better patient outcomes when their care is evidence-based and worse when it is not, and (in the preceding paragraphs) audits showing that the majority of interventions can be evidence-based in a wide variety of specialties and settings. Since the publication of the first edition of this book, the question is no longer *whether* to teach and practice EBM, but *how* to do so most effectively and efficiently. Accordingly, the next few paragraphs will summarize evidence on strategies for teaching its elements. If the preceding chapters have had any impact you might start by generating some three- or four-part questions about learning, practicing and teaching EBM.

Who are the "patients"?

Who are the "patients" or "population" representing the subjects in our questions? Two groups may be readily identified: the clinicians who use EBM and the patients they care for. There is an accumulating body of evidence relating to the impact of EBM on students and health care professionals. This ranges from systematic reviews and randomized controlled trials of training in the skills of EBM through to cohort studies and some qualitative research describing the experience of EBM practitioners. There is less evidence about the effect of EBM on patient care or patients' perceptions of their care, but the latter aspect is now being addressed as part of the growing interest in "evidence-based patient choice".

What is the intervention (and the control maneuver)?

One reason why studies of the ultimate effect of teaching the elements of EBM are difficult to conduct is that it is unethical to generate a comparison group of clinicians who are allowed to become out of date and ignorant of life-saving evidence accessible to, and known by, the evidence-based clinicians in the experimental group. Similarly, clinicians will not take kindly to being assigned to an evidence-poor teaching intervention. For example, when one school allocated its students to a traditional or an innovative EBM-style pathway (problem-based, self-directed, etc.), the students voted with their feet, abandoned the traditional program, and destroyed the "experiment".

In many studies of the impact of EBM teaching, the "intervention" has proved difficult to define. In some, it is an approach to clinical practice whilst in others it is training in one of the discrete "microskills" of EBM such as MEDLINE searching or critical appraisal. Given the pervasive nature of EBM, it seems likely that attempts to teach a single aspect of EBM are likely to be "contaminated" by exposure to the whole EBM package. Moreover, evaluating EBM strategies in clinical environments ill-suited (by tradition or active hostility) to their practice is likely to underestimate their effect. Although it is not difficult to conceive of the changes in resources and timetabling that would promote the introduction of EBM into undergraduate and postgraduate learning, the challenge is to precede these changes with solid evidence that they will work. Although this challenge has rarely been set or met by previous architects of new curricula, we nonetheless have sought it here.

What are the relevant outcomes?

Effective EBM interventions will produce a wide range of outcomes. Changes in clinicians' knowledge and skills are relatively easy to detect and demonstrate. Changes in their behaviors and attitudes are harder to confirm. And, for the reasons already stated, randomized trials employing hard clinical outcomes are unethical. Accordingly, studies demonstrating better patient survival when practice is evidence-based (and worse when it is not) are limited to the cohort "outcomes research" studies described in this book's Introduction.

1. Effects of teaching strategies on searching skills

A randomized trial among first clinical year medical students in Oxford showed that a 3-hour session on question formulation and database searching produced significant gains in the quality of evidence retrieved.[1] The failure of control students to gain these skills by "diffusion" means that these skills must be formally learnt, confirming an earlier cohort study.[2] EBM journal clubs have been shown to change reading habits.[3]

2. Effects of teaching strategies on critical appraisal skills

The use of educational prescriptions, and their completion in the form of CATs, as part of a clinical teaching package has been shown to be popular and effective.[4] A cohort study compared clinical trainees exposed to weekly conferences that stressed critical appraisal with an unexposed group, and then crossed them over. Although the gains in clinical epidemiology skills were statistically significant, they were small and the authors stressed the need for more effective teaching of these skills.[5] The need to integrate critical appraisal training into direct patient care was shown in two before–after studies that documented various changes in objective tests of critical appraisal knowledge[6] and in the ability to appraise original research articles,[7] but no increase in the use of the medical literature in writing up patient notes or in time spent reading.

3. Effects of teaching strategies on clinical decision-making

An undergraduate program adopting problem-based, self-directed learning around diagnosis and therapy[8] has been shown to result in clerks making more and better clinical decisions, which they are better able to defend than peers educated in a more conventional program, and this effect has been shown to persist up to 15 years after graduation.[9] A systematic review of randomized trials of postgraduate training methods intended to improve performance found that traditional didactic teaching methods are ineffective but that EBM approaches are successful.[10] Two non-systematic reviews[11, 12] concluded that knowledge gains among undergraduates are consistent but among postgraduates are small. A subsequent systematic review, now in press, found that the optimal methods for teaching critical appraisal include the use of a small-group, needs-assessed format, with support and facilitation over the long term, to impart knowledge and skills (the similarities between this list and our advice in Ch. 8 is not coincidental!). In that review, undergraduates learned more readily than postgraduates did, but it concluded that there is good evidence that knowledge and skills can be taught.

Reports describing evidence-based rejuvenations of traditional educational events are burgeoning, and case reports and a survey of US residency programs[15] have concluded that the determinants of continuing high attendance at postgraduate journal clubs are mandatory attendance, the teaching of critical appraisal skills, emphasizing the primary literature, independence from faculty, and (of course) free food! Finally, qualitative research has confirmed that teaching and learning critical appraisal are enjoyable, a fact that should not be underestimated in one's working life!

For those of you who have read this far, that's it! We hope you have enjoyed this book and its accompanying resources as well as learned from them, and we would appreciate your suggestions on how to make them more useful as well as more enjoyable.

Cheers.

References

1   Rosenberg et al 1999 J Royal Coll Phys
2   Bull Med Libr Assoc 1992; 80: 23–8.
3   JAMA 1988; 260: 2537–41.
4   Ann Roy Soc Phys Surg Can 1995; 28: 396–8.
5   J Gen Int Med 1989; 4: 384–7.
6   J Gen Intern Med 1994; 9: 436–9.
7   J Gen Int Med 1991; 6: 330–4.
8   JAMA 1987; 257: 2541–4.
9   Can Med Assoc J 1993; 148: 969–76.
10 Int J Psychiatry Med 1998; 28: 21–39.
11 Can Med Assn J 1993; 148: 945–52.
12 Can Med Assn J. 1998; 158: 177–81.
13 Arch Intern Med 1995; 155: 1193–7.

Appendix 1: Confidence intervals*

What does the "confidence interval" (CI) tell us? The CI gives a measure of the precision (or uncertainty) of study results for making inferences about the population of all such patients. A strictly correct definition of a 95% CI is, somewhat opaquely, that 95% of such intervals will contain the true population value. Little is lost by the less pure interpretation of the CI as the range of values within which we can be 95% sure that the population value lies. The CI approach places a clear emphasis on quantification, in direct contrast to the P values which arise from the significance testing approach. The P value is not an estimate of any quantity but rather a measure of the strength of evidence against the null hypothesis of "no effect". The P value by itself tells us nothing about the size of a difference, nor even the direction of that difference. P values on their own are thus not informative in papers or abstracts. By contrast, CIs indicate the strength of evidence about quantities of direct interest, such as treatment benefit.[1-3] They are thus of particular relevance to practitioners of evidence-based medicine.

The estimation approach to statistical analysis exemplified in the CI aims to quantify the effect of interest (the sensitivity of a diagnostic test, the rate of a prognostic event, the NNT for a treatment, etc.) and also to quantify the uncertainty in this effect. Most often this is a range of values either side of the estimate in which we can be 95% sure that the true value lies. The convention of using the value of 95% is arbitrary, just as is that of taking $P < 0.05$ as being significant, and authors sometimes use 90 or 99% CIs. Note that the word "interval" means a range of values and is thus singular. The two values that define the interval are called "confidence limits".

---

* Prepared for this book by Douglas G Altman of the ICRF Medical Statistics Group and the Centre for Statistics in Medicine, Oxford, UK.

The CI is based on the idea that the same study carried out on different samples of patients would not yield identical results, but their results would be spread around the true but unknown value. The CI estimates this "sampling variation". In most circumstances, the CI is calculated from the observed estimate of the quantity of interest, such as the difference (d) between two proportions, and the standard error (SE) of the estimate for this difference. A 95% CI is obtained here as $d \pm 1.96SE$ (The formula will vary according to the nature of the outcome measure and the coverage of the CI, but it will be of this general type). Table A.1 gives the structure of the SEs for some clinical measurements of interest. For example, in a randomized placebo-controlled trial of acellular pertussis vaccine,[4] 72/1670 (4.3%) infants developed pertussis among those receiving the vaccine and 240/1665 (14.4%) did so among the control group. The difference in percentages, known as the absolute risk reduction (ARR), is 10.1%. The SE of this difference is 0.99%, so that the 95% CI is $10.1 \pm 1.96 \times 0.99\%$, and therefore runs from 8.2 to 12.0%.

Despite the considerably different philosophical approaches, CIs and significance tests are closely related mathematically. Thus a "significant" P value of $P < 0.05$ will correspond to a 95% CI which excludes the value indicating equality; for example, this value is 0 for the difference between two means or proportions and 1 for a relative risk or odds ratio. (The equivalence of the two approaches may not be exact in some circumstances.) The prevailing view is that estimation, including CIs, is the preferable approach to summarizing the results of a study, but CIs and P values are complementary and many papers use both.

The uncertainty (imprecision) expressed by a CI is to a large extent affected by the square root of the sample size. Small samples provide less information than large ones, and the CI is correspondingly wider in a smaller sample. For example, a paper comparing the characteristics of three tests to diagnose *H. pylori*[5] reported the sensitivity of the ^{14}C urea breath test as 95.8% (95% CI, 75–100%). While the figure of 95.8% is impressive, the small sample of 24 adults with *H. pylori* means that there is considerable uncertainty in that estimate

Table A.1 Standard errors (SEs) and confidence intervals (CIs) for some clinical measures of interest

Clinical measure	Standard error (SE)	Typical calculation of SE and CI[a]

I. THERAPEUTIC STUDIES

(a) Outcome is an event – one group

In general, r events are observed among n patients, so the observed proportion is p = r/n. In the illustrative example, p = 24/60 = 0.4 (or 40%).

Proportion **(event rate in one group)**	$SE = \sqrt{\dfrac{p \times (1-p)}{n}}$ where p is proportion and n is number of patients	If p = 24/60 = 0.4 (or 40%): $SE = \sqrt{\dfrac{0.4 \times 0.6}{60}} = 0.063$ (or 6.3%) 95% CI is 40% ± 1.96 × 6.3%, i.e. 276 to 52.4%[b]

(b) Outcome is an event – comparison of two groups[c]

In general, r_1 and r_2 events are observed among n_1 and n_2 patients in two groups, so the observed proportions are $p_1 = r_1/n_1$ and $p_2 = r_2/n_2$.
In the illustrative example, $p_1 = 15/125$ (or 12%) and $p_2 = 30/120 = 0.25$ (or 25%)[d].

Absolute risk reduction (ARR)	$SE = \sqrt{\dfrac{p_1(1-p_1)}{n_1} + \dfrac{p_2(1-p_2)}{n_2}}$	$ARR = p_2 - p_1 = 0.13$ (or 13%): $SE = \sqrt{\dfrac{0.12 \times 0.88}{125} + \dfrac{0.25 \times 0.75}{120}} = 0.049$ (or 4.9%) 95% CI is 13% ± 1.96 × 4.9%, i.e. 3.4 to 22.6%[b]

Table A.1 *(cont'd)*

Clinical measure	Standard error (SE)	Typical calculation of SE and CI[a]
Number needed to treat (NNT)	Not calculated	NNT = 100/ARR = 100/13 = 7.7 CI is obtained as reciprocal of CI for ARR, so 95% CI is 100/22.6 to 100/3.4 or 4.4 to 29.4[e]
Relative risk (RR)	$RR = p_1/p_2$ $SE \text{ of } \log_e RR = \sqrt{\dfrac{1}{r_1} + \dfrac{1}{r_2} - \dfrac{1}{n_1} - \dfrac{1}{n_2}}$	$RR = 0.12/0.25 = 0.48$ (48%); $\log(RR) = -0.734$ $SE \text{ of } \log_e RR = \sqrt{\dfrac{1}{15} + \dfrac{1}{30} - \dfrac{1}{125} - \dfrac{1}{120}} = 0.289$ 95% CI for $\log_e RR$ is $-0.734 \pm 1.96 \times 0.289$, i.e. -1.301 to -0.167; 95% CI for RR is 0.272 to 0.846 or 27.2 to 84.6%
Relative risk reduction (RRR)	Not calculated	$RRR = 1 - RR = 1 - p_2/p_1 = 1 - 12/25 = 0.52$ (or 52%). 95% CI for RRR is obtained by subtracting CI for RR from 1 (or 100%), i.e. 0.154 to 0.728 or 15.4 to 72.8%

Table A.1 *(cont'd)*

Odds ratio (OR)

$$OR = \frac{r_1(n_2 - r_2)}{r_2(n_1 - r_1)}$$

$$OR = \frac{15 \times 90}{30 \times 110} = 0.409; \log_e OR = -0.894$$

$$SE \text{ of } \log_e OR = \sqrt{\frac{1}{r_1} + \frac{1}{r_2} - \frac{1}{n_1 - r_1} - \frac{1}{n_2 - r_2}}$$

$$SE \text{ of } \log_e OR = \sqrt{\frac{1}{15} + \frac{1}{30} + \frac{1}{90} + \frac{1}{110}} = 0.347$$

95% CI for $\log_e OR$ is $-0.894 \pm 1.96 \times 0.347$, or -1.573 to -0.214; 95% CI for OR is 0.207 to 0.807

(c) Outcome is a measurement

Mean

If s is the standard deviation (SD) of n observations, SE = $s/\sqrt{n}$

95% CI is mean $\pm t \times SE^f$

If mean = 17.2, s = 6.4, n = 38, then SE = $6.4/\sqrt{38}$ = 1.038 and 95% CI is $17.2 \pm 2.026 \times 1.038$ or 15.1 to 19.3

Difference between two means[b]

If s_1 and s_2 are SDs of n_1 and n_2 observations, SE(diff) =

$$\sqrt{\frac{(n_1-1)s_1^2 + (n_2-1)s_2^2}{n_1+n_2-2} \times \left(\frac{1}{n_1} + \frac{1}{n_2}\right)}$$

95% CI is mean diff $\pm t \times SE(diff)^f$

If $mean_1$ = 17.2, s_1 = 6.4, n_1 = 38, $mean_2$ = 15.9, s_2 = 5.6, n_2 = 45, then mean difference = $17.2 - 15.9 = 1.3$,

$$SE(diff) = \sqrt{\frac{37 \times 6.4^2 + 44 \times 5.6^2}{38+45-2} \times \left(\frac{1}{38} + \frac{1}{45}\right)} = 1.317$$

and 95% CI is $1.3 \pm 1.99 \times 1.317$ or -1.32 to 3.92

Table A-1 (cont'd)

Clinical measure	Standard error (SE)	Typical calculation of SE and CI[a]
II. DIAGNOSTIC STUDIES *(a) A single proportion*	In general, r diagnoses are observed among n patients, so the observed proportion is p = r/n. Using the notation of Chapter 3, the sensitivity is a/(a + b), the positive predictive value is a/(a + c) the specificity is b/(b + d) and the negative predictive value is d/(c + d). The illustrative example is from Table 3.5. The sensitivity is 731/809 = 90% or 0.90, and the specificity is 1500/1770 = 85% or 0.85. p = 73/82 = 0.89 (or 89%)	
Sensitivity, specificity, predictive values	$$SE = \sqrt{\frac{p \times (1-p)}{n}}$$ where p is proportion and n is number of patients	For the sensitivity, p = 731/809 = 0.90 (or 90%): $$SE = \sqrt{\frac{0.90 \times 0.10}{809}} = 0.0105 \text{ (or } 1.05\%)$$ 95% CI is 90% ± 1.96 × 1.05% or 87.9 to 92.1%[b]

Table A.1 (cont'd)

(b) Likelihood ratio

In general, the likelihood ratios for positive or negative test results are, respectively, obtained as either LR+ = sensitivity/(1 − specificity) or LR− = (1 − sensitivity)/specificity.

Likelihood ratio (LR)	
$LR+ = [a/(a + c)]/[c/(b + d)]$	$LR+ = (731/809)/(270/1770) = 0.9/(1 − 0.85) = 6.0$
	$\log_e(LR+) = 1.792$
$LR− = [c/(a + c)]/[b/(b + d)]$	
$SE \text{ of } \log_e LR+ = \sqrt{\dfrac{1}{a} + \dfrac{1}{b} - \dfrac{1}{a+c} - \dfrac{1}{b+d}}$	$SE \text{ of } \log_e RR = \sqrt{\dfrac{1}{731} + \dfrac{1}{1500} - \dfrac{1}{809} - \dfrac{1}{1770}} = 0.0153$
	95% CI for $\log_e LR+$ is $1.792 \pm 1.96 \times 0.0153$,
	i.e. 1.762 to 1.822
	95% CI for LR+ is 5.82 to 6.18
	A similar approach is used to derive a CI for LR−

[a] In general, a confidence interval is obtained by taking the estimate of interest and adding and subtracting a multiple of the SE. Except in the case of means or differences in means, the multiple is taken as a value from the standard normal distribution. For a 95% CI, the multiplier is 1.96; for a 90% CI it is 1.645, and for a 99% CI it is 2.576. For proportions this method is the traditional method referred to in footnote "b". In some cases, such as for RR (and RRR) and OR, the CI is obtained for the logarithm of the quantity of interest and the values are antilogged (logs to base e are used in the table).

Table A.1 *(cont'd)*

[b] The method illustrated is the traditional method. It works fine in most cases but is not recommended when sample sizes are small and/or proportions are near either 0% or 100% (in which case it is possible for the CI to include impossible values outside the range 0–100%). Newer methods are recommended both for general use and especially for the circumstances described. The methods are too complex to include here – they are described in reference 9 and incorporated into the software included with it.

[c] As used in this book, p_1 corresponds to the event rate in the experimental group (EER) and p_2 to the event rate in the control group (CER).

[d] The above calculations assume that comparisons are between two independent groups. For CIs derived from paired data (e.g. from crossover trials or matched case–control studies), and also CIs for some other statistics, see references 8 and 9.

[e] When the ARR is not significantly different from zero, one limit of the 95% CI is negative. Taking reciprocals gives a CI for the NNT with one negative value, which corresponds to a harmful effect. We can write the CI in terms of both the NNT and NNH. For example, a 95% CI for the ARR of −5% to 25% gives the 95% CI for the NNT of 10 as −20 to 4 or from NNH = 20 to NNT=4. However, the values included in this interval are NNH from 20 to ∞ (infinity) and NNT from 4 to ∞. We can write this as NNH = 20 to ∞ to NNT = 4 (see references 9 and 10).

[f] For the calculation of a CI for a mean or the difference between means, the multiplier referred to in footnote "a" for a 95% CI is not 1.96 but a value from the t distribution.

as shown by the wide CI. If the same sensitivity had been observed in a sample of 240, the 95% CI would have been from 92.5 to 98.0%. (Note that in this example the CI was not obtained using the traditional method shown in Table A.1. See footnote b for an explanation.)

In randomized trials, non-significant results (i.e. those with $P > 0.05$) are especially prone to misinterpretation. CIs are especially useful here as they show whether the data are compatible with clinically useful true effects. For example, one of the outcomes in a randomized trial to compare suturing and stapling for large-bowel anastomosis[6] was wound infection, which occurred in 10.9 and 13.5% of cases, respectively ($P = 0.30$). The 95% CI for this difference of 2.6% is -2% to $+8\%$. Even in this study of 652 patients there thus remains the possibility that there is a modest difference in wound infection rates for the two procedures. In a smaller study, uncertainty is greater. Sung et al[7] carried out a randomized trial to compare octreotide infusion and emergency sclerotherapy for acute variceal hemorrhage in 100 patients. The observed rates of controlled bleeding were 84% in the octreotide group and 90% in the sclerotherapy group, giving $P = 0.56$. Note that the figures for uncontrolled bleeding are similar to those for wound infection in the study just considered. In this case, however, the 95% CI for the treatment difference of 6% is -7% to $+19\%$. This interval is very wide in relation to the 5% difference that was of interest. It is clear that the study cannot rule out a large difference in effectiveness, so that the authors' conclusion that "octreotide infusion and sclerotherapy are equally effective in controlling variceal haemorrhage" is certainly not valid. When, as here, the 95% CI for the absolute risk reduction (ARR) spans zero, the CI for the NNT is rather peculiar. The NNT and its CI are obtained by taking reciprocals of the ARR values (and multiplying by 100 when those values are given as percentages). Here we get NNT $= 100/6 = 16.6$ with a 95% CI -14.3 to 5.3. As noted in footnote "e" of Table A.1, this CI represents values of NNT from 5.3 to infinity and NNH from 14.3 to infinity.

CIs can be constructed for most common statistical estimates or comparisons.[8,9] For RCTs, these include differences between means or proportions, relative risks, odds ratios, and the number needed to treat (NNT). Likewise, CIs can be obtained for all the main estimates arising in studies of diagnosis – sensitivity, specificity, positive predictive value (all of which are simple proportions) and likelihood ratios – and estimates derived from meta-analyses and case–control studies. A computer program for personal computers which covers many of these methods is available with the second edition of *Statistics with Confidence*.[9]

While CIs are desirable for the primary results of a study; they are not needed for all results. Further, it is important that, when given, they relate to the contrast of interest. In particular, when two groups are compared, the appropriate CI is that for the difference between the groups, as illustrated in the above examples. Not only is it unhelpful to give separate CIs for the estimates in each group, but this presentation can be quite misleading. When the authors have not provided CIs, these can often be constructed using the results provided in their paper.

The most appropriate methods of statistical analysis and presentation must be largely a matter for personal judgement, although increasingly journals are requesting or requiring authors to use CIs when presenting their key findings. It seems clear that the wide adoption of CIs in medical research papers over the last decade has been of great benefit to a more correct understanding of the external evidence used in the practice of evidence-based medicine.

References

1   Gardner M J, Altman D G. Confidence intervals rather than P values: estimation rather than hypothesis testing. BMJ 1986; 292: 746–50.

2   Rothman K J, Yankauer A. Confidence intervals vs. significance tests: quantitative interpretation. Am J Public Health 1986; 76: 587–8.

3   Bulpitt C J. Confidence intervals. Lancet 1986; 1: 494–7.

4   Trollfors B, Taranger J, Lagergard T et al. A placebo-controlled trial of a pertussis-toxoid vaccine. N Eng J Med 1995; 333: 1045–50.

5   Fallone C A, Mitchell A, Paterson W G. Determination of test performance of less costly methods of *Helicobacter pylori* detection. Clin Invest Med 1995; 18: 177–85.

6 Docherty J G, McGregor J R, Akyol A M, Murray G D, Galloway D J. Comparison of manually constructed and stapled anastomoses in colorectal surgery. Ann Surg 1995; 221: 176–84.

7 Sung J J Y, Chung S C S, Lai C-W et al. Octreotide infusion or emergency sclerotherapy for variceal haemorrhage. Lancet 1993; 342: 637–41.

8 Gardner M J, Altman DG (eds). Statistics with confidence. British Medical Journal, London, 1989.

9 Altman D G, Machin D, Bryant T N, Gardner M J (eds). Statistics with confidence. 2nd edn. British Medical Journal, London, 2000 (including CIA software).

10 Altman D G. Confidence intervals for the number needed to treat. BMJ 1998; 317: 1309–12.

Appendix 2: Glossary

Terms you are likely to encounter in your clinical reading

Absolute risk reduction (ARR). See **treatment effects**.

Case–control study. A study which involves identifying patients who have the outcome of interest (cases) and control patients without the same outcome, and looking back to see if they had the exposure of interest.

Case series. A report on a series of patients with an outcome of interest. No control group is involved.

Clinical practice guideline. A systematically developed statement designed to assist clinician and patient decisions about appropriate health care for specific clinical circumstances.

Cohort study. Involves identification of two groups (cohorts) of patients, one which received the exposure of interest, and one which did not, and following these cohorts forward for the outcome of interest.

Confidence interval (CI). Quantifies the uncertainty in measurement. It is usually reported as 95% CI, which is the range of values within which we can be 95% sure that the true value for the whole population lies. For example, for an NNT of 10 with a 95% CI of 5–15, we would have 95% confidence that the true NNT value was between 5 and 15.

Control event rate (CER). See **treatment effects**.

Cost–benefit analysis. Assesses whether the cost of an intervention is worth the benefit by measuring both in the same units; monetary units are usually used.

Cost-effectiveness analysis. Measures the net cost of providing a service as well as the outcomes obtained. Outcomes are reported in a single unit of measurement.

Cost minimization analysis. If health effects are known to be equal, only costs are analyzed and the least costly alternative is chosen.

Cost–utility analysis. Converts effects into personal preferences (or utilities) and describes how much it costs for some additional quality gain (e.g. cost per additional quality-adjusted life-year, or QALY).

Crossover study design. The administration of two or more experimental therapies one after the other in a specified or random order to the same group of patients.

Cross-sectional study. The observation of a defined population at a single point in time or time interval. Exposure and outcome are determined simultaneously.

Decision analysis (or clinical decision analysis). The application of explicit, quantitative methods that quantify prognoses, treatment effects, and patient values in order to analyze a decision under conditions of uncertainty.

Ecological survey. A survey based on aggregated data for some population as it exists at some point or points in time; to investigate the relationship of an exposure to a known or presumed risk factor for a specified outcome.

Event rate. The proportion of patients in a group in whom the event is observed. Thus, if out of 100 patients, the event is observed in 27, the event rate is 0.27. Control event rate (CER) and experimental event rate (EER) are used to refer to this in control and experimental groups of patients, respectively. The patient expected event rate (PEER) refers to the rate of events we'd expect in a patient who received no treatment or conventional treatment. See **treatment effects**.

Evidence-based health care. Extends the application of the principles of evidence-based medicine (see below) to all professions associated with health care, including purchasing and management.

Evidence-based medicine. The conscientious, explicit and judicious use of current best evidence in making decisions about the care of individual patients. The practice of evidence-based medicine means integrating individual clinical expertise with the best available external clinical evidence from systematic research

Experimental event rate (EER). See **treatment effects**.

Incidence. The proportion of new cases of the target disorder in the population at risk during a specified time interval.

Inception cohort. A group of patients who are assembled near the onset of the target disorder.

Intention-to-treat analysis. A method of analysis for randomized trials in which all patients randomly assigned to one of the treatments are analyzed together, regardless of whether or not they completed or received that treatment.

Likelihood ratio (LR). The likelihood that a given test result would be expected in a patient with the target disorder compared with the likelihood that that same result would be expected in a patient without the target disorder.

Calculation of sensitivity/specificity/LR

	Disease positive	Disease negative
Test positive	a	b
Test negative	c	d

Sensitivity = $a/(a + c)$

LR+ = [sensitivity/(1 − specificity)] = $[a/(a + c)] \div [b/(b + d)]$

Specificity = $d/(b + d)$

LR− = (1 − sensitivity)/specificity = $[c/(a + c)] \div [d/(b + d)]$

Positive predictive value = $a/(a + b)$, negative predictive value = $d/(c + d)$

Pre-test probability = $(a + c)/(a + b + c + d)$

Meta-analysis. A systematic review that uses quantitative methods to summarize the results.

N-of-1 trials. In such trials, the patient undergoes pairs of treatment periods organized so that one period involves the use of the experimental treatment and the other involves the use of an alternate or placebo therapy. The patient and physician are blinded, if possible, and outcomes are monitored. Treatment periods are replicated until the clinician and patient are convinced that the treatments are definitely different or definitely not different.

Negative predictive value. Proportion of people with a negative test who are free of the target disorder. See also **likelihood ratio**.

Number needed to treat (NNT). The inverse of the absolute risk reduction and the number of patients that need to be treated to prevent one bad outcome. See **treatment effects**.

Odds. A ratio of the number of people incurring an event to the number of people who have non-events.

Odds ratio (OR). The ratio of the odds of having the target disorder in the experimental group relative to the odds in favor of having the target disorder in the control group (in cohort studies or systematic reviews) or the odds in favor of being exposed in subjects with the target disorder divided by the odds in favor of being exposed in control subjects (without the target disorder).

Calculations of OR/RR for use of trimethoprim-sulfamethoxazole prophylaxis in cirrhosis

	Adverse event occurs (infectious complication)	Adverse event does not occur (no infectious complication)	Totals
Exposed to treatment (experimental)	1 a	b 29	a+b 30
Not exposed to treatment (control)	c 9	d 21	c+d 30
Totals	10 a+c	b+d 50	a+b+c+d 60

CER = c/(c+d) = 0.30

EER = a/(a+b) = 0.033

Control event odds = c/d = 0.43

Experimental event odds = a/b = 0.034

Relative risk = EER/CER = 0.11

Relative odds = odds ratio = (a/b)/(c/d) = ad/bc = 0.08

Patient expected event rate. See **treatment effects**.

Overview. See **systematic review**.

Positive predictive value. Proportion of people with a positive test who have the target disorder. See also **likelihood ratio**.

Post-test odds. The odds that the patient has the target disorder after the test is carried out (pre-test odds × likelihood ratio).

Post-test probability. The proportion of patients with that particular test result who have the target disorder (post-test odds/[1 + post-test odds]).

Pre-test odds. The odds that the patient has the target disorder before the test is carried out (pre-test probability/ [1 – pre-test probability]).

Pre-test probability/prevalence. The proportion of people with the target disorder in the population at risk at a specific time (point prevalence) or time interval (period prevalence) See also **likelihood ratio**.

Randomization (or random allocation). Method analogous to tossing a coin to assign patients to treatment groups (the experimental treatment is assigned if the coin lands "heads" and a conventional, "control" or "placebo" treatment is given if the coin lands "tails").

Randomized controlled clinical trial (RCT). A group of patients is randomized into an experimental group and a control group. These groups are followed up for the variables/outcomes of interest.

Relative risk reduction (RRR). See **treatment effects**.

Risk ratio (RR). The ratio of risk in the treated group (EER) to risk in the control group (CER) – used in randomized trials and cohort studies: RR = ERR/CER.

Sensitivity. Proportion of people with the target disorder who have a positive test. It is used to assist in assessing and selecting a diagnostic test/sign/symptom. See also **likelihood ratio**.

SnNout. When a sign/test/symptom has a high **S**e**n**sitivity, a **N**egative result rules **out** the diagnosis. For example, the sensitivity of a history of ankle swelling for diagnosing ascites is 93%; therefore if a person does not have a history of ankle swelling, it is highly unlikely that the person has ascites.

Specificity. Proportion of people without the target disorder who have a negative test. It is used to assist in assessing and selecting a diagnostic test/sign/symptom. See also **likelihood ratio**.

SpPin. When a sign/test/symptom has a high **Sp**ecificity, a **P**ositive result rules **in** the diagnosis. For example, the specificity of a fluid wave for diagnosing ascites is 92%; therefore if a person does have a fluid wave, it rules in the diagnosis of ascites.

Systematic review. A summary of the medical literature that uses explicit methods to perform a thorough literature search and critical appraisal of individual studies and that uses appropriate statistical techniques to combine these valid studies.

Treatment effects. The evidence-based journals journals (*Evidence Based Medicine* and *ACP Journal Club*) have achieved consensus on some terms they use to describe both the good and bad effects of therapy. We will bring them to life with a synthesis of three randomized trials in diabetes which individually showed that several years of intensive insulin therapy reduced the proportion of patients with worsening retinopathy to 13% from 38%, raised the proportion of patients with satisfactory hemoglobin A1c levels to 60% from about 30%, and increased the proportion of patients with at least one episode of symptomatic hypoglycemia to 57% from 23%. Note that in each case the first number constitutes the "experimental event rate" (EER) and the second number the "control event rate" (CER). We will use the following terms and calculations to describe these effects of treatment:

When the experimental treatment reduces the probability of a bad outcome (worsening diabetic retinopathy)

RRR (relative risk reduction). The proportional reduction in rates of bad outcomes between experimental and control participants in a trial, calculated as |EER − CER|/CER, and accompanied by a 95% confidence interval (CI). In the case of worsening diabetic retinopathy, |EER − CER|/CER = |13% − 38%|/38% = 66%.

ARR (absolute risk reduction). The absolute arithmetic difference in rates of bad outcomes between experimental and control participants in a trial, calculated as |EER − CER|, and accompanied by a 95% CI. In this case, |EER − CER| =|13% − 38%| = 25%.

NNT (number needed to treat). The number of patients who need to be treated to achieve one additional favorable outcome, calculated as 1/ARR and accompanied by a 95% CI. In this case, 1/ARR = 1/25% = 4.

Calculations for the occurrence of diabetic retinopathy in IDDMs

Occurrence of diabetic retinopathy at 5 years among insulin-dependent diabetics in the DCCT trial		Relative risk reduction (RRR)	Absolute risk reduction (ARR)	Number needed to treat (NNT)
Usual insulin regimen (CER)	Intensive insulin regimen (EER)	$\dfrac{\text{|EER − CER|}}{\text{CER}}$	|EER − CER|	1/ARR
38%	13%	|13% − 38%|/ 38% = 66%	|13% − 38%| =25%	1/25% = 4 pts, for 6 years, with intensive insulin Rx

When the experimental treatment increases the probability of a good outcome (satisfactory hemoglobin A1c levels)

RBI (relative benefit increase). The proportional increase in rates of good outcomes between experimental and control patients in a trial, calculated as |EER − CER|/CER, and accompanied by a 95% confidence interval (CI). In the case of satisfactory hemoglobin A1c levels, |EER − CER|/CER =|60% − 30%|/30% = 100%.

ABI (absolute benefit increase). The absolute arithmetic difference in rates of good outcomes between experimental and control patients in a trial, calculated as |EER – CER|, and accompanied by a 95% confidence interval (CI). In the case of satisfactory hemoglobin A1c levels, |EER – CER| = |60% – 30%| =30%

NNT (number needed to treat). The number of patients who need to be treated to achieve one additional good outcome, calculated as 1/ARR and accompanied by a 95% CI. In this case, 1/ARR = 1/30% = 3.

When the experimental treatment increase the probability of a bad outcome (episodes of hypoglycemia)

RRI (relative risk increase). The proportional increase in rates of bad outcomes between experimental and control patients in a trial, calculated as |EER – CER|/CER, and accompanied by a 95% confidence interval (CI). In the case of hypoglycemic episodes, |EER – CER|/CER = |57% – 23%|/23% = 148%. (RRI is also used in assessing the impact of "risk factors" for disease.)

ARI (absolute risk increase). The absolute arithmetic difference in rates of bad outcomes between experimental and control patients in a trial, calculated as |EER – CER|, and accompanied by a 95% confidence interval (CI). In the case of hypoglycemic episodes, |EER – CER| = |57% – 23%| = 34%. (ARI is also used in assessing the impact of "risk factors" for disease.)

NNH (number needed to harm). The number of patients who, if they received the experimental treatment, would lead to one additional patient being harmed, compared with patients who received the control treatment, calculated as 1/ARR and accompanied by a 95% CI. In this case, 1/ARR = 1/34% = 3.

Index

Page numbers in **bold** type refer to figures; those in *italics* to tables.

absolute benefit increase (ABI) 113, 251–2
absolute risk increase (ARI) 113, 252
absolute risk reduction (ARR) *112*, 113, 251
academic half days 199–201
American College of Physicians (ACP)
 ACP Journal Club 34, 60, 109
 Clinical Efficacy Assessment Program 59
Aidsline 32
anemia, iron deficiency 72–8, *73*, 89
aneurysms, abdominal aortic 95
angina, unstable 4, 116
angiotensin-converting enzyme (ACE) inhibitors 44
antihypertensive therapy 44–6
antioxidants 37, 47–51
applied health research 8
appraisal 4–5, 169
 critical *see* critical appraisal
aspirin 7, 119, 141, 147
 poisoning 4
atenolol 45
atrial fibrillation 98–9, 124, 139–41, 146–7
audit
 clinical services 6
 preventive care 39–40, 57–9

bargains 180
barriers 180

beliefs 179
best case scenario 97
best evidence 1
 finding current 29–63
 keeping up to date 29
 resources 29–63
Best Evidence 4, 32–3
 antioxidants 48
 carotid stenosis 51
 diabetes and hypertension 43–4, 46
 ulcerative colitis 56
beta-blockers 7, 44
beta-carotene 37, 47–51
Bioethicsline 32
BioMedNet 33
BMJ website 46
burden of illness 179

calcium antagonists 155–68
Canadian Task Force on the Periodic Health Examination 40, 92, 172
Cancerlit 32
cardiovascular disease 37, 47–51
carotid bruit 37
carotid stenosis 38, 51–3, 116
carotid surgery 7
carotid ultrasound 38, 51–3
case-control studies 158–9, 245
case-finding 88–90
case reports 159
CATs (critically appraised topics) 25, 186
 diagnostic tests 87–8
 hypertension and calcium antagonists 168
 inpatient setting 191, 192
 iron deficiency in elderly 89

CATs *(cont'd)*
  learning and teaching 87–8
  multiple sclerosis and
    interferon 130
  outpatient clinics 195, 198
  therapy 105
CD, organization 9–11
chance nodes 140
clinical decision analysis (CDA)
  123, 138–44, 246
  applicability 143–4
  importance 142–3
  sensitivity analysis 142
  validity 141–2
clinical decision making
  support systems 35
  teaching strategies 231–2
Clinical Evidence 31, 41, 47, 63
clinical expertise 1
  and pre-test probability 82
clinical issues *19*
*Clinical Journal of Sport
  Medicine* 60
Clinical Medicine (Kumar and
  Clark, 3rd edition) 47, 54
clinical prediction guides
  diagnostic tests 71, 80
  prognosis 100
clinical questions *see* questions
clinical skills 8
clinical trials *see* trials; trials,
  randomized controlled
clinicians
  audit 6
  EBM practice 3–6
  limitations 7
Cochrane Clinical Trials Registry
  46
Cochrane Database of Systematic
  Reviews 32, 46
Cochrane Library 32–3, 41,
  46, 62
Cochrane Reviews 4
cognitive dissonance 18
cognitive resonance 18

cohort studies 157–8
communication skills 8
compliance 131–3
  low 132
  non-compliance, causes 132
  trials 109
computers
  clinical decision support
    systems 35
  reminder systems 39–40,
    57–9
  searching ability 43
confidence intervals 5, 163,
  233–42, 245
  number needed to treat 118
  prognosis 102
consent 87
consistency 160
continuing professional
  development, self-evaluation
  228–9
control event rate (CER) 111,
  112, 120–21, 136
cost-benefit analysis 147, 245
cost-effectiveness analysis 147, 245
cost minimization analysis 146,
  245
cost-utility analysis 147, 246
critical appraisal
  diagnostic tests 67–87
  evaluation 222–3
  pre-test probabilities 83
  teaching strategies 231
Critical Care 34
critically appraised topics
  see CATs
crossover study design 246
cross-sectional study 246
current awareness 43, 59–62
Current Contents 34

databanks 134
databases 32–3
  local/regional/national practice
  82–3

dechallenge-rechallenge study 160
decision analysis *see* clinical decision analysis
decision trees 139–40
derivation sets 99
diabetes mellitus and hypertension 35–6, 42–7
diagnostic tests 67–93
  accuracy 80–81, *81*
  affordability 80–81, *81*
  application 80–87
  availability 80–81, *81*
  CATs 87–8
  clinical prediction guides 71, 80
  clinical research 1
  clusters of diagnostic features *see* clinical prediction guides
  consequences 87
  critical appraisal 67–87
  independence 86–7
  independent blind comparisons *68*, 68–70
  likelihood ratios *see* likelihood ratios
  multiple 80
  outcomes 91
  patient spectrum *68*, 70
  post-test probability 72–4, *73*, *78*, 84–7, 249
  precision 80–81, *81*
  pre-test probability 72–4, *73*, 82–4, *83*, **84**, *85*, 249
  reference (gold) standard *68*, 68–71
  sensitivity 72–4, *73*
  sensitivity analysis 81
  specificity 72–4, *73*
  survival 91, 93
  teaching 92–3
  test-treatment threshold *81*, **84**, 84–7
  validation in independent group of patients *68*, 71
  validity 67–80, *68*

dose-response gradient 160
dyspnea 13–14

EBM
  definition 1, 7–8
  evaluation 219–32
  interest in 1–3
  limitations 7–8
  modes/styles of practice 4–5
  outcomes 6–7, 230–32
  practice of 3–6
  pseudo-limitations 7–8
  realizations 2
  recent developments 3
  teaching methods 183–218
  uses 8
ecological survey 246
economic analyses 144–50
  importance 148
  applicability 149–50
  validity 145–7
education, professional 8
  see also learning; teaching
  obsolescence 29
  self-evaluation 228–9
educational closure 187
educational prescriptions 23–7, **24**, *26–7*, 186
EMBASE 44
enalapril 45
ethics 7
evaluation
  critical appraisal 222–3
  evidence-based medicine 219–32
  question-asking 219–22
  research 22
  searching 220–22
  teaching 207
event rate 246
Evidence-Based Cardiology 32
Evidence-Based Cardiovascular Medicine 34, 60
Evidence-Based Health Care Policy and Practice 34

Evidence-Based Health Policy and Management 60
evidence-based medicine *see* EBM
Evidence-Based Medicine 34, 60, 109
Evidence-Based Medicine Reviews (EBMR) 32, 41, 43-5, 58, 62
Evidence-Based Mental Health 32, 34, 60
Evidence-Based Nursing 32, 34, 60
Evidence-Based on Call 31, 172
experimental event rate (EER) 111, *112*, 246

Family Practice JC (POEMS) 34
follow-up *see* patient follow-up

grand rounds 201-2
group sessions (academic half days) 199-201
guidelines 169-81
  applicability 178-81
  behavior changes 181
  components 170-2, *171*
  development groups 181
  evidence component 170, *171*
  instructional component 170, *171*
  killer Bs 170, 178-181, *179*
  levels of evidence 172, *173-7*
  screening *91*
  as systematically developed statements 170
  validity 172-8

harm 155-67
  applicability of studies 165-6
  importance of studies 161-5
  labeling 90, 92
  from therapy 120-23
  validity of studies 155-61

Harrison's Principles of Internal Medicine CD-ROM 47
Harrison's textbook 31, 54, 57
health care by post code 180
Healthstar 32
heparin 116
home remedies 48
hypertension 116, 117
  antihypertensive therapy 44-6
  calcium antagonists 155-68
  diabetes mellitus 35-6, 42-7
  labeling 90
  transient ischemic attack 37-8
hypertext 43

inception cohort 96, 247
information resources 29-63
informed consent 87
intention-to-treat analysis 109-10, 247
interferon therapy 105, 107, 109, 111, 121-3, 125-31
Internet 43
  home remedies 48
  Ovid service 44
iron deficiency anemia 72-8, *73*, 89

journal clubs 198-9
Journal of Pediatrics 60
journals
  evidence-based/online 34
  hand-searching 134
  subscribing to 33-4
  summary 34, 60-62
  validity criteria 60-62, *61*

keeping up to date 29
knowledge
  background 15-18
  foreground 15-18

labeling 90, 92
league tables 148, *148-9*

learning
  see also education,
    professional; teaching
  common issues *213–14*
  counterproductive behaviors
    215–17
  critically appraised topics
    (CATs) 87–8
  for deep understanding
    184–5
  discussions *211–12*
  general notions 183–7
  ground rules *208–9*
  healthy climate *211*
  lifelong 8
  multi-staged 187
  outpatient clinics 193–8
  planning activities *209–11*
  preparation for using EBM
    skills *217–18*
  problem-based (learning by
    inquiry) 29
  about teaching 207, *208–18*
  time management *212–13*
lectures 202–4
leukemia, chronic lymphocytic
  95
librarians 186
likelihood of being helped vs.
  harmed (LHH) 124–9, 166
likelihood ratios 247
  diagnostic tests 72–4, *73*
  multilevel 76–80, *77*, *78*
  nomogram 78, **79**
limitations
  pseudo-limitations 7–8
  universal 7

MEDLINE 32, 33, 44, 62
  antioxidants 49
  carotid stenosis 52–3
  diabetes and hypertension
    45–6
  high-sensitivity searches *50*
  medlineplus 48

  search filters 49
  ulcerative colitis 57
mentors 207
meta-analyses 133, 247
multiple sclerosis 105, 107, 111,
  121–3, 125–31
myocardial infarction
  routines 169
  therapeutic trials 7

National Guideline
  Clearinghouse 59
negative predictive value *73*, 248
Neurosurgery 34
n-of-1 trials 150–53, 247
normality, definitions 69–70
number needed to harm (NNH)
  116, 120–23, 127–9, *137*,
  163–6, 252
number needed to treat (NNT)
  5, *112*, 113–18, *114–15*,
  120–23, 127–9, *137*, 248,
  251, 252
  confidence intervals 118
  nomogram **122**

odds ratios (ORs) 136, *137*, 248
  adverse events 161–5
  sensitivity analysis 163
opportunity costs 145, 180
organization, book/CD 9–11
outcomes
  diagnostic tests 91
  evidence-based medicine 6–7,
    230–32
  harm studies 160–61
  likelihood over time 100–101
  objective criteria 98
  patient follow-up *see* patient
    follow-up
  and patient preferences 124
  patient samples 96
  prognosis 98
  research 7
  screening 91

outpatient clinics 193–8
Ovid 44
Oxford Textbook of Medicine
47, 54

pathophysiology 161
patient follow-up
  adverse events 159–60
  presentation *194*
  prognosis 96–8
  randomized trials 108–9
  rounds 195–8, *196*
patient presentations *26–7, 194*
patient's expected event rate
  (PEER) 120–21, 127, 136,
  163–6
patients
  behavior 181
  beliefs 179–80
  evidence-based patient choice
    229
  expectations 123–9
  exposed vs. non-exposed
    157–8
  informed consent 87
  labeling 90, 92
  outcomes *see* outcomes
  preferences 124–5, 127, 166,
    179–80
  questions 21–2
  randomization 106–8, 249
  samples 96
  subgroups 98–100
patients' values 1, 179–80
  self-evaluation 223–7
  treatment 123–9
Peds Journal Club 34
pharmacists 186
placebo 106
pneumonia 15–16
positive predictive value *73*, 249
post-test probability 72–4, *73,
  78*, 84–7, 249
pre-test probability 72–4, *73*,
  82–4, *83*, **84**, *85*, 249

prevalence statistics,
  regional/national 82
preventive care audit 39–40,
  57–9
problem-based learning 29
problem-solving resources
  59–62
prognosis 95–103
  application to patients 102–3
  clinical prediction guides 100
  confidence intervals 102
  importance 100–102
  objective outcome criteria 98
  patient follow-up 96–8
  patient samples 96
  patient subgroups 98–100
  precision 101–2
  questions about 95
  sensitivity analysis 97–8
  survival 91, 93
  survival curves 100–101, **101**
  test set 98–100
  validity 95–103, *95*
PubMed Clinical Queries
  carotid stenosis 52
  related articles 51
  search filters 49–51
  ulcerative colitis 55–6

quality-adjusted life-years
  (QALYs) 140, 143, 147, 148
quality of life 91
questions 13–27
  about prognosis 95
  asking, evaluating performance
    219–22
  background 15–18, **17**
  foreground 15–18, **17**
  learner-centered 22
  patient-based 22
  patients' 21–2
  posing answerable 20–21
  students' 15
  teaching asking of *22–7, 23*,
    219–20

well-built *15*
where/how they arise 18–20

randomized trials *see* trials,
    randomized controlled
rating scales 124–5, **125**
reference (gold) standards *68*,
    68–71
relative benefit increase (RBI)
    111, 251
relative risk increase (RRI) 252
relative risk reduction (RRR)
    111–13, *112*, 250–51
relative risks (RRs) 136
    of adverse event 161–5
replication 5, 169
research
    action research 22
    clinically relevant *see* best
        evidence
    diagnostic tests 1
    evaluation 22
    outcomes 7
    qualitative 21–2, 129–31
    systematic reviews *see*
        systematic reviews
rounds 187–93
    ambulatory morning report
        197
    consultant walking rounds
        189, 192
    dead time *190*, 193
    follow-up visits 195–8, *196*
    grand rounds 201–2
    morning report *188*, 191
    post-take (admission) 187–91,
        188
    preceptorship during follow-up
        visits *196*
    pre-clinic conferences 195, *196*
    pure education *190*, 193
    review card rounds *189*,
        192–3
    social issues *189*, 193
    work rounds *188*, 191–2

Scientific American Medicine
    (*SAM*) 31
    diabetes and hypertension 47
    preventive healthcare 59
    ulcerative colitis 55, 57
screening 67, 88–90
    false-positive results 90
    guidelines *91*
    outcomes 91
search engines 30
search filters 49–51
searching 5, 35–63, 169–70
    basic steps 41–59
    evaluation 220–22
    general search strategy **42**
    skills development 7
    teaching strategies 250–31
self-evaluation 219–29
sensitivity 249
    diagnostic tests 72–4, *73*
sensitivity analysis
    clinical decision analyses 142
    diagnostic tests 81
    odds ratios/relative risk 163
    prognosis 97–8
severity factor 129
SHARR 34
Silverplatter 34
SnNout 74, *75*, 249–50
specificity 250
    diagnostic tests 72–4, *73*
spontaneous bacterial peritonitis
    204
SpPins 74, *75*, 250
stroke 7
    prognostic factors 98–9
summary journals 34, 60–62
survival 91, 93
survival curves 100–101, **101**
systematic reviews 105, 133–8,
    250
    applicability 138
    evidence-driven 171
    free-standing 171
    heterogeneity 135

systematic reviews *(cont'd)*
  as highest level of evidence
    155–6
  importance 136–8
  language 135, 172
  necessity-driven 59, 171
  publication bias 172
  qualitatively similar results 135
  quantitatively identical results
    135
  validity 134–6

teaching
  see also education,
    professional; learning
  active/interactive 184–5
  clinical decision-making
    231–2
  clinical settings 185–6
  critical appraisal strategies
    231
  critically appraised topics
    (CATs) 87–8
  criticism 207
  diagnostic tests 92–3
  evaluation 207
  general notions 183–7
  in-patient service 187–93
  learner-centred 184
  learning about 207, *208–18*
  methods 183–218
  mistakes 204–7
  modeling 185
  outpatient clinics 193–8
  patient-centred 184
  preparation 186
  question-asking *22–7, 23,*
    219–20
  rounds *see* rounds
  searching skills 230–31
  self-evaluation 227–8
  slow/long 184
  small 186
  strategies, evaluation *229–32*
  workshops 186, 207

temporal arteritis 4
test-treatment threshold *81*, **84**,
  84–7
tests sets (validation sets) 99
textbooks
  obsolescence 62–3
  traditional 30–32
therapy 105–53
  alternative treatments 166
  critically appraised topics 105
  decision trees 139–40
  effects 250
  feasibility 119–20
  harmful 120–23
  magnitude of treatment effect
    111–17
  patient's preferences 124–5,
    127, 166, 179–80
  patient's values/expectations
    123–9
  placebo 106
  qualitative differences in
    response 119, *120*
  randomized trials *see* trials,
    randomized
  reports 105–29
  risks and benefits 120–23,
    126, 165–6
thromboembolism, venous 4
time management *212–13*
training sets (derivation sets) 99
transient ischemic attack 37–8,
  51–3, 119
treatment *see* therapy
trials
  n-of-1 150–53, 247
  negative 134–5
  systematic reviews *see*
    systematic reviews
trials, randomized controlled
  249
  adverse events 156–7
  applicability 118–29
  compliance 109
  concealed randomization 107

double-blind method 110
false-negative results 107, 108
false-positive results 107, 108
importance 110–18
intention-to-treat analysis
109–10, 247
overview 105
patient follow-up 108–9
random allocation 106–8,
249
validity 106–10
worst case analysis 109

UK Prospective Diabetes Study
45, 46, 47
ulcerative colitis 39, 53–7
ultrasound, carotid 38, 51–3
UpToDate 31, 63
antioxidants 49
carotid stenosis 51
diabetes and hypertension 47

US National Library of Medicine
33, 48, 62
utilities 140, 142, 144, 147

validation sets 99
validity
diagnostic tests 67–80, *68*
guidelines 172–8
harm studies 155–61
journals 60–62, *61*
prognosis 95–103, *95*
randomized trials 106–10
systematic reviews 134–6
videotapes 203
virtual libraries 8
vitamin E 37, 47–51

warfarin 7, 124, 147
website 10–11
workshops 186, 207
worst case scenario 97